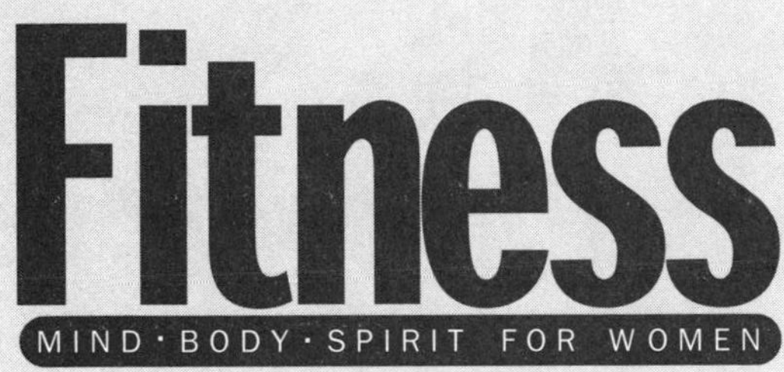

STRETCHING

Fitness

MIND · BODY · SPIRIT FOR WOMEN

S T R E T

EDITORS OF *FITNESS* MAGAZINE

WITH KAREN ANDES

THREE RIVERS PRESS

NEW YORK

C H I N G

AUTHOR'S NOTE: THIS BOOK PROPOSES A PROGRAM OF PHYSICAL EXERCISE FOR THE READER TO FOLLOW. HOWEVER, BEFORE STARTING THIS OR ANY OTHER EXERCISE PROGRAM, YOU SHOULD CONSULT YOUR PHYSICIAN.

PUBLISHED BY THREE RIVERS PRESS, 201 EAST 50TH STREET, NEW YORK, NEW YORK 10022.
MEMBER OF THE CROWN PUBLISHING GROUP.

RANDOM HOUSE, INC. NEW YORK, TORONTO, LONDON, SYDNEY, AUCKLAND
WWW.RANDOMHOUSE.COM

PRINTED IN THE UNITED STATES OF AMERICA
DESIGN BY LAUREN MONCHIK

CREDITS

FOR ROUNDTABLE PRESS:
DIRECTORS: JULIE MERBERG, MARSHA MELNICK, SUSAN E. MEYER
PROJECT EDITOR: MEREDITH WOLF SCHIZER
ILLUSTRATOR: JUDY FRANCIS
FOR *FITNESS* MAGAZINE:
EDITOR-IN-CHIEF: SARAH MAHONEY
FITNESS DIRECTOR: MARTICA HEANER
FITNESS EDITOR: JANET LEE
LICENSING MANAGER: TAMMY PALAZZO

LIBRARY OF CONGRESS CATALOGING-IN-PUBLICATION DATA
FITNESS STRETCHING / EDITORS OF FITNESS MAGAZINE WITH KAREN ANDES.
1. STRETCHING EXERCISES. I. ANDES, KAREN. II. FITNESS (NEW YORK, N.Y.)
RA781.63.F55 2000
613.7'1—dc21 99-35413
CIP

ISBN 0-609-80160-0

10 9 8 7 6 5 4 3 2

ALSO BY THE EDITORS OF *FITNESS* MAGAZINE

THE COMPLETE BOOK OF FITNESS

PREGNANCY FITNESS

C O N T

E N T S

ACKNOWLEDGMENTS

The authors would like to acknowledge the American College of Sports Medicine and The American Council on Exercise for their continued dedication to providing research findings and education, so that educators in this field can improve the quality of life for others. In addition, the authors would like to thank the authors listed in the Bibliography, whose books enriched this one, and the staff of *Fitness* magazine.

WHY STRETCH?

EVERYONE KNOWS THAT STRETCHING FEELS GOOD. SO WHY DO SO MANY OF US PUT IT AT THE BOTTOM OF OUR FITNESS LIST? WHY DO WE INVEST SO MUCH TIME IN THE WORKOUTS THAT'LL MAKE US *LOOK* GOOD, BUT PUT SO LITTLE TIME INTO THOSE THAT MAKE US *FEEL* GOOD AND FUNCTION BETTER? THOSE OF US WHO BOTHER TO STRETCH AT ALL TEND TO THROW IN A FEW STRETCHES *BEFORE* A WORKOUT (NOT THE BEST TIME TO STRETCH—ALTHOUGH THERE'S STILL SOME DEBATE ABOUT THIS) AND THEN, IF THERE'S ENERGY AND TIME, DO A FEW MORE STRETCHES AT THE END. STRETCHING IS LIKE THE NEGLECTED MIDDLE CHILD IN THE "FITNESS FAMILY"; IT IS JUST AS IMPORTANT AS THE TWO OTHER SIBLINGS—CARDIOVASCULAR CONDITIONING AND STRENGTH TRAINING. AND THE OLDER WE GET, THE MORE IMPORTANT STRETCHING BECOMES.

The 1980s marked the decade of aerobic exercise. We jogged and jumped our way toward cardiovascular health. The 1990s were the decade of strength. We lifted our way toward stronger muscles and bones, greater muscle definition, and a healthier muscle-to-fat ratio. Now, as we enter into a whole new century, stretching may be the activity of choice, especially for more "mature" individuals whose old "war wounds" from overzealous or uninformed fitness regimens or aches from years of inactivity are causing pain and cramping lifestyles. Even people with no pains to heal are taking up stretching because it offers a "kinder, gentler workout." The question is, is it enough to keep you fit?

Before we launch into this book and tout the many valid wonders of stretching, we want to say up front that stretching by itself won't make you totally fit—just as aerobics or strength training alone won't either. We promote a balanced approach to fitness, one that meets all the body's needs; the body needs endurance (both cardiovascular and muscular), strength, and flexibility. But since this book is about stretching, we'll assume that you already know how to meet those other needs—or will look elsewhere for that information (such as *The Complete Book of Fitness*). Perhaps *because* stretching has been the neglected middle child of fitness, we think it deserves a book of its own.

Stretching isn't flashy, and contrary to what some stretching and yoga classes proclaim, it won't make you lean or superbuff. But it *will* lengthen your muscles, lubricate your joints, rebalance your nervous system, refresh a weary body, and calm a worried mind. Of all three obvious dimensions of fitness, we think stretching is the simplest (it doesn't require special equipment) and most pleasurable (it feels good) but also the most humbling (many of us are very tight). It is also one of the safest ways to exercise, and you can do it anywhere.

Unfortunately, much conflicting information has been published about the best ways to stretch. Even many stretching "experts" disagree on how to do it. So, although the act of stretching is simple, the philosophies about how to stretch are anything but.

We've sorted through all that information so that you don't have to, and we have arrived at some sensible conclusions. We'll share with you the hows, whys, and whens of stretching; fill in all the little details that make the difference between a so-so stretch and a wonderful one; and give you appropriate stretches to match your sports, your job, your gender, and your life.

First, Let's Define Stretching: Five Ways to Stretch

Technically there are five different ways to stretch.

1. Static stretching is a held posture. You take the muscle just up to (but not beyond) the point of tightness and hold that position for 10 seconds to a minute. (We recommend 10 to 30 seconds, according to the American College of Sports Medicine [ACSM] stretch guidelines listed in the next chapter.) All the stretches in this book are static, which means this is a *passive* activity. You shouldn't work hard to increase your flexibility but rather should "surrender" into it. Otherwise, you will defeat the purpose of the stretch. Many forms of yoga simply string together a series of static stretches, some held longer than others. Static stretching is one of the safest, least invasive forms of exercise, and you can do it anywhere!

2. Ballistic stretching is usually thought of as a bouncing stretch and is a big no-no, banned from the fitness industry in the 1980s. Bouncing while stretching (like in those old Canadian Air Force exercises where you bounce down to touch your toes) will actually give you results opposite those you seek. When you bounce, your muscles stretch suddenly and violently like a rubber band being yanked (when you do that to a rubber band, it can break). Likewise, ballistic stretching can damage both the muscles and the joints. The body, in its wisdom, protects itself against ballistic stretching with something known as the "stretch reflex." When the body senses potentially violent motion, the muscles tighten to protect the threatened joint—and this happens just when you're trying to stretch. (A good example of the stretch reflex at work is when you nod off to sleep in the middle of a boring meeting or class and your head drops and bobs back up.) Ballistic stretching isn't all bad, however. Many sports involve ballistic movements; a gymnast leaping in the air to do a split is performing a ballistic stretch, and so is a martial artist delivering a forceful kick. Ballistic stretches take a tremendous amount of energy and coordination to perform, and even well-conditioned athletes get injured doing these things. But the average person who stretches for health almost never needs to do ballistic stretches.

3. Active stretching is stretching while in motion, usually through a joint's full range of motion. Whenever you move, especially through a full range, one set of muscles stretches while its opposing group contracts. For instance, weight-training exercises like squats, bench presses, and lunges are active stretches (regardless of whether you do these motions with extra resistance). In a bench press, for instance, as you *lower* the weight, the chest muscles stretch and the back muscles contract. As you *lift* the weight, the chest contracts and the back muscles stretch. Many of the larger movements used in an aerobics class are active stretches as well. It's important to warm up before performing active stretches, especially when you add extra weight or resistance. Five minutes of gentle, rhythmic motions like walking or an aerobic warm-up make the muscles and joints more pliable for active stretches.

4. Passive stretching is partner-assisted stretching. Like the name implies, during a passive stretch you let an outside force—your partner—push your stretches slightly beyond the point where you'd go alone. You have to know what you're doing here so that you never force a stretch into a dangerous position. (Overstretching, after all, has often been used as a form of torture. The medieval torture device known as the rack was passive stretching to the extreme.)

If you're going to do this, you and your partner must maintain good communication, stretch slowly, and be familiar with the sensible boundaries of a stretch. One disadvantage of passive stretching is that your muscles don't really learn or retain the information of how to get into those deeper stretches. When you do your stretches alone, however, your body learns how to make the stretch movement itself.

5. PNF, or Proprioceptive Neuromuscular Facilitation, is a fancy term for tensing and then relaxing a muscle. PNF stretching was designed by physical therapists and physicians and usually involves first tensing the muscle and then having someone assist the stretch. Some fitness instructors teach simple PNF stretches in class. For instance, they'll have you hold the back of your head and push your head into your hands in an isometric contraction to tense the neck muscles, then pull your head forward to stretch the back of the neck. Theoretically, fatiguing a muscle before stretching it will tire the muscle out so it will be more willing to slide into a deeper stretch. But PNF is a fairly complicated venture, best overseen by a therapist and not recommended for anyone with high blood pressure or coronary artery disease. It can also be uncomfortable, since not everyone enjoys the tensing part of the exercise.

What Does Stretching Do?

▪ It keeps you from turning into a little old person before your time.

Since you probably don't spend much time hanging upside down like a bat to counteract gravity, the force of gravity tends to work on you over time. Thus, you're at risk for falling into bad postural habits. If you also spend a lot of time sitting, your "slouch patterns" get more extreme. This creates a vicious cycle. When your body hurts, you don't want to move, and then inertia makes the problem worse. Your body adapts to inertia by making your muscles shorter and tighter. Stretching corrects the problem. It lengthens muscles, soothes painful joints, and often changes your relationship to gravity (which can soothe "hot" or "trouble" spots in your joints by sending nourishing blood into otherwise neglected areas). Walking, riding a bike, and lifting weights can make you feel better temporarily and "loosen up" your joints, but these things also make your muscles tighter. (After exercise, muscles go into a healing phase in which they shorten and tighten.) The only way to correct this situation is by stretching regularly.

■ It helps you relax.

To lengthen a muscle, you have to relax it. When you stretch, you consciously inform your muscles to "progressively relax." This mind-body activity is an art unto itself requiring concentration and skill. Stretching reduces the amount of electrical "firing" inside the muscle, which tells it to stay tight. Releasing tension has many health benefits, including lower blood pressure, improved circulation, minimized pain and fatigue, and a speedier disposal of waste products (like lactic acid) from the muscles. Lengthened, relaxed muscles also absorb nutrients more easily and then they use that energy more efficiently.

■ It feels good and is good for you.

As obvious as this sounds, the pleasurable aspect of stretching is a big selling point. It's hard to make this same claim about a bench press or the twenty-third mile of a marathon. When you stretch, certain "stretch receptors" located in and next to your muscles tell your brain that you're relaxed and feel good. The brain responds by sending chemicals of well-being (such as endorphins and serotonin) to the muscles and into the nervous system. Therefore, stretching reinforces positive moods. Of course, stretching isn't all pleasure. It often rides that delicate border between pleasure and pain. But the mind perceives it differently the longer you do it. So if you're new to stretching and you're moaning through your first few classes, hang in there; not only will you get looser over time, you'll learn to like it more!

■ It sends blood (and the nutrients carried in the blood) to your joints.

Improved circulation keeps joints healthy and makes your muscles and connective tissues (the ones that attach muscle to muscle and muscle to bone) more elastic and, therefore, less likely to get injured. Connective tissue, by nature, isn't very elastic. So when you overstretch it, it tends to stay that way for life. This makes your joints wobbly, makes you less coordinated, and puts you at risk for injury and arthritis. You're actually better off breaking a bone than overstretching connective tissue, since bones can repair themselves.

■ It keeps your joints well lubed.

Stretching sends a fresh batch of synovial fluid into your joints. Synovial fluid pads and protects the joints from injury. When you don't stretch or move, the fluid turns thick and sludgy, like oil in a car that hasn't been driven in a while. A healthy dose of synovial fluid gives extra cushioning to the joints, creating more freedom of movement. The lack of fluid makes joints "dry" and "creaky" and speeds up joint deterioration. A little old lady taking small cautious steps, for instance, doesn't have a healthy amount of synovial fluid in her hips. A lifetime of stretching can keep a walking stride youthful and long.

■ It improves your posture and balance.

Bad habits like slouching or always carrying a bag on the same side add up over time and create bad posture, which can leave you lopsided and prone to injuries. Stretching helps you "retrain" and realign your posture, but for this it usually works best in conjunction with strength exercise. For instance, if you have rounded shoulders and sunken chest, your chest muscles are tight and your upper-back muscles are stretched and weak. To correct the imbalance, strengthen your upper back and stretch your chest.

■ It minimizes suffering from lower-back pain.

If you sit for too long or exercise without stretching (always shortening muscles with contractions without lengthening them with stretches), you create the perfect atmosphere for back pain. The lower-back muscles tend to stay tight and contracted unless you move or stretch them (and the abdominals stay weak and don't support the torso). The hamstrings (back of the leg), hip flexors (front of the hip), and other muscles attached to the pelvis get tight and weak, or can even atrophy, and therefore cause stress to the lower back. Many nerves run through the lower back and pelvic area, so tight muscles in these places also constrict nerve function. No painkiller in the world can actually fix the *cause* of this problem—only stretching can.

Some Gray Areas

▪ Does stretching reduce soreness after a workout?

One to three days after a workout, muscles often feel tender to the touch. This phenomenon (known as Delayed Onset Muscle Soreness, or DOMS) is caused by muscle fibers rebuilding themselves after getting "broken down" while exercising. Some early research (documented in *Science of Flexibility* by Michael J. Alter) reported that stretching reduces DOMS. This was based on the theory that tight muscles are associated with soreness. Tight muscles hold on to metabolic wastes longer than loose ones do. While recent research hasn't been able to prove without a doubt that this is true, the ACSM's inclusion of stretching in its general recommendations at least supports the importance of stretching for maintaining fitness. Common sense and experience can also tell you that stretching a muscle makes it longer, looser, more flexible, and less sore.

▪ Does stretching aid injury prevention?

The jury is still out regarding the role stretching plays in injury prevention. Logic dictates that if a joint has a bigger, pain-free range of motion, then it can perform better and won't move as quickly into a tight, dangerous "don't go there" zone; therefore, it will be less likely to get injured. Tight muscles also contribute to joint injuries.

For instance, a tight thigh muscle puts extra stress on the knee joint, which then causes instability and pain. A tight shoulder muscle compresses the sensitive soft tissue in the shoulder and leaves the shoulder joint unstable and sore. When one joint is tight or painful, not only is that joint more vulnerable to injury but several joints are, since joints are strung together like links on a chain. Pull one and they're all affected. (That's why if you hurt your knee you can feel pain in your ankle or hip.) Then again, there's no scientific evidence to back up the claim that stretching—before or after exercise—reduces injuries. In fact, a 1994 study from the University of Hawaii examined 1,500 marathon runners and found that those who stretched actually had *higher* rates of injury. While that was just one isolated study, the lack of scientific data in support of stretching has caused some health professionals to dismiss it as overrated or a waste of time. Ultimately, you have to trust your own experience. When do *you* feel or perform better—when you are tight or loose? You don't need a scientific study to tell you how you feel. Plenty of other scientific studies say that stretching the right way for the right amount of time is good for you, although there's still no hard data on its role in injury prevention. At the very least, if you *think* that stretching prevents injuries, then it just might (our motto is, if the placebo works, take it). If you stretch correctly, it can't hurt you. Stretching is one of the most risk-free forms of exercise you can do.

■ Does stretching make you stronger?

Well, that depends on how you stretch. Technically, if you just do static stretches, no. Muscles need to work against resistance (e.g., weights, elastic bands, or water) through a "full range of motion" (see below) for approximately 8 to 15 repetitions (to fatigue or failure) in order to get stronger. Muscles also get stronger through endurance activities like walking or biking, although not as strong as with resistance training. Many yoga and stretch classes bill themselves as gentler ways to get strong. And yes, if you're moving fairly quickly from posture to posture, combining active and static stretches, you'll get some strength benefits because your muscles are moving against resistance. Your body weight supplies the resistance—called *isotonic* resistance. When you hold *static* stretches, your muscles go into *isometric* contractions. (Push your palms together. That's isometric. The joints don't move.) Of all the muscle contractions there are, isometrics are the least effective for building strength, and muscles aren't as strong in isometric contraction as when moving. (Muscles are strongest when you move or lower a weight with gravity—an *eccentric* contraction. Muscles are next strongest when lifting a weight against gravity, a *concentric* contraction.) When performing static postures, you employ isometric contractions to hold your body still. But the main muscles that work around a joint tend not to get much stronger in these positions because they don't move through a full range of motion. So if you're taking a yoga or stretch class to get *stronger*, you have to analyze its routines and movements to see if the class combines active stretches that move joints through a full range of motion as well as static stretches. If it doesn't, then probably you're not going to get significantly stronger. But you may get stretched!

■ What's all this about "full range of motion"?

You may hear this phrase a lot, but people tend to misunderstand it. If you raise your arm and swing it around, you should be able to move it comfortably in all directions, unless you've had a shoulder injury (which minimizes your range of motion). You may have also seen people freely swing their arms in many directions with weights in their hands. This is not a good thing. Just because your arm *can* go through impressively large ranges of motion, doesn't mean it *should* (especially with added resistance). A more accurate phrase to describe this would be "effective range of motion." When you use weights or extra resistance, you should be conservative and only take the weights through the "effective" range of motion that will work the muscle without compromising the joint. The same is true when you stretch. Just because your arm or leg can move in all kinds of positions doesn't mean it *should*. You should move a joint only as far as it needs to go to give the muscles a sufficient stretch—and you should *never force a stretch* or put pressure on a joint, especially when it hurts! As with weight training, when you stretch, there are effective ranges of motion—and there are danger zones. More about that in the next chapter.

What Stretching *Won't* Do for You

- **It won't give you a good warm-up.**

Stretching doesn't increase the core temperature of your muscles (only gentle aerobic activity like brisk walking does that). Therefore, it's not a good warm-up. If you like to stretch before you work out (and many people do), do your stretches *after* a 3- to 5-minute "aerobic" warm-up but before the main body of your workout. More about this in the next chapter.

- **It won't help you shed body fat.**

Some rigorous yoga classes maintain ongoing movements that make you sweat, raise your heart rate, and burn fat. But the *continuous motions* make it aerobic. Stretching does not. Holding stretches won't melt fat or burn huge amounts of calories (maybe a few more than if you were sitting still, but not a significant amount). To burn fat you need to add three to five 20- to 60-minute cardiovascular workouts per week to your routine. Two sessions of strength training per week will also improve your muscle-to-fat ratio (which speeds metabolism and spurs fat loss). But since time is an issue, many people flock to classes that provide a cardiovascular, strength, and flexibility workout in a one-stop shop (a perfectly valid way to train, as long as you get what's promised!).

Why Am I So Tight and What Can I Do About It?

Flexibility refers to the degree of movement you have around a particular joint. When you can move a limb in all directions through a "normal" range of motion, you're flexible. Trying to become so flexible you could get a job as a contortionist in the circus overstretches your connective tissue, which, you now know, leaves your joints vulnerable to arthritis and injury. Some people, however, are simply more flexible than others. Children are more flexible than adults, and women are more flexible than men. (Women have a wider pelvis for childbearing, which allows the muscles in the hips and lower back to move with greater ease. Women's connective tissue also loosens up to prepare for giving birth. Perhaps this makes it generally more elastic as well. [See "Stretching During Pregnancy," page 191.]) Ultimately, how flexible you are depends on many factors:

Genetics

We're all put together differently. Length and elasticity of muscles and connective tissue (tendons and ligaments) are genetically determined, as is the structure of a joint. Some people have looser connective tissue and bigger "joint sockets." But just because you're flexible in one joint doesn't necessarily mean you'll be flexible in another. Each joint is different, though stretching offers equal-opportunity-healing medicine for all joints.

Age

It's certainly no secret that the older we get, the tighter we get, although just how much this changes depends to a large extent on our levels of activity and the ways we use our muscles. We reach the peak of our flexibility between the ages of six and twelve. Our flexibility starts to level off in adolescence, and once we hit twenty-five, it's all downhill from there. If we don't use it, we definitely lose it. As we get older, the tiny strands of connective tissue inside our muscles tend to shorten (creating a nasty form of "shrinkage" called Adaptive Muscle Shortening, or AMS). Unless we keep our muscles strong with activity, the muscles atrophy. Instead of firm "lean beef" under our skin, we have more fat, and our muscles become denser with collagen fibers in our connective tissue. Collagen is a protein in abundant supply that our bodies use for making living tissue. It's strong but hardly flexible at all. This makes our muscles tighter and weaker. Age also changes the way the muscle fibers "communicate" with one another (through something called cross-links.) When we're young, our cross-link communication is fairly direct. As we get older the cross-links get more complicated, so the "messages" meet more resistance as they travel through the various pathways. The result? Decreased performance. As we get older, we tend to get more dehydrated as well, especially in our tendons. Joints also "dry up" (less movement means less protective synovial fluid). All of this reduces the muscles' ability to stretch and makes the tendons more rigid. Sounds glum, to be sure. The most certain way to exacerbate this problem is to sit around all day! Only a regular stretching regimen can help you out of this mess.

Injury

When you're injured and can't move a limb for a long time, the muscles, connective tissues, and joints lose their ability to stretch. Since connective tissue and joints have only minimal stretching capabilities to begin with, decreased motion can seriously affect your ability to move. A gentle stretching program can restore mobility to various degrees, depending on the severity of the injury.

Balanced muscles

If you've ever spotted a bodybuilder with huge thighs but flat, ill-defined hamstrings, you can bet he or she has tight hamstrings and will probably develop knee and hip pain if it isn't present already. Muscles work best in pairs—both to strengthen and to relax the body.

The problem is, people tend to develop their muscles in a lopsided way, favoring the "showy" muscles they see in the mirror over the humble supporting ones, usually on the back side. So there are lots of folks out there hobbling around with big chests but weak upper backs, strong abdominals but weak lower backs, "quadzilla" thighs but invisible hamstrings. The flashy overdeveloped muscles tug too hard on one side of the body while the neglected muscles stay weak. First one joint is affected, then several. Over time, the body starts to act like the leaning tower of Pisa, until it gradually gets pulled severely out of alignment. In both your stretching and your strength workouts you should aim for equal strength and flexibility in muscle pairs and try to even out your lopsidedness before continuing with the same old bad habits, which might make things worse. If one side of your leg or torso, for example, is significantly stronger than the other, strengthen the weak side and stretch the tight side to bring them into balance. Once you're better balanced, *then* you can update your strength and stretch program. (A certified personal trainer or physical therapist can help you determine where you're off balance.)

Does strength training make you "muscle-bound"?

First of all, "muscle-bound" is an old term, born during the Charles Atlas era of strength training. ("Ninety-pound weaklings" who got sand kicked in their faces by big "he-men" could then follow Charles Atlas's mail-order course to become even more muscular than the bullies.) Guys who defended the right to be "ninety-pound weaklings" and, later, misinformed coaches came up with the "muscle-bound" theory, and it stuck. Wielding a dumbbell doesn't make you so absurdly tight your muscles turn into a coat of armor. Yes, it's true that you can still spot an occasional "muscle-bound" bodybuilder whose forearms can't touch his sides. But he didn't get that way from lifting. He got that way by *not stretching*. You can be both strong and loose, but you have to stretch as often as you lift.

Strength training puts muscles into a constant state of repair. The muscle tissue gets "broken down" during training and on the following days repairs itself with food and rest. Recuperating muscles feel slightly sore and tight to the touch because they're armoring themselves against further invasion. (Recovering muscles don't like to be interrupted with more hard work—but gentle activity is fine!) Muscles end up in a constantly shortened state—which is a passive form of contraction. While sitting all day doesn't work your muscles, it doesn't stretch them either. Muscles shortened through inactivity waste energy. They act like your car engine idling at a higher speed. You burn fuel but don't go anywhere! Tight muscles therefore don't have as much reserve strength. Tight muscles also put constant pressure on nearby joints, so the poor joints never get a chance to rest (and, like everything else in the body, they need rest). Imagine this scenario: someone you know (not you, of course) strength trains like a maniac two or three days a week, doesn't stretch, and on the other days sits around all day. So that person takes the tightness from training and compounds that with the tightness from inactivity and experiences tightness times two! Eventually, if he or she keeps this up as years go by, this perpetual tightness will break down the cartilage in the joints (very painful and immobilizing).

What Happens to Muscles and Tendons During a Stretch?

Muscles contain sensitive "stretch receptors," which tell the nervous system if the body is tight or relaxed—and the nervous system reacts accordingly (stimulating the release of adrenaline when we're stressed or more pleasurable neurotransmitters like serotonin or endorphins when we're feeling good). All of this happens on a cellular level. There are two types of sensory receptors, the muscle spindle and the Golgi tendon organ. (Don't go to sleep on us yet. We promise not to get too technical.) The muscle spindle exists *inside* the muscle and basically determines the extent to which the muscle is going to stretch or contract (based on how much force is being exerted against it). The Golgi tendon organ sits in the space where the muscles meet the tendons and oversees the stretchability of the muscles and tendons. (These stretch receptors also rush in like good soldiers to protect the muscles and tendons with the "stretch reflex" when a stretch becomes too sudden or violent.)

Temporary vs. Lasting Changes

For all your stretching, you're going to get two types of results. One is temporary, or elastic. The muscles act like a spring. They stretch for a little while and then return to their original length. Short bouts of stretching create these temporary changes. But you can also make permanent, or plastic, changes.

To do this, you have to create the right conditions for permanent change and make sure your muscles are warm before you stretch. (Your muscles should be about 1 to 3 degrees warmer than normal—like they are during aerobic exercise.) Heat makes muscles more elastic. (Warm muscles can stretch to 1.6 times their resting length. Body heat also alters the structure of the collagen fibers, giving them a bit more flexibility.) You need to hold each stretch for 10 to 30 seconds, as we describe in "Stretching 101," and you have to do this on a *regular basis*—2 or 3 days per week, or a little every day informally. Your body will adapt to all this stretching by increasing the flexibility of both muscles and joints—so keep it up.

A Brief History of Yoga and Stretching

Ancient yogis would probably be amused at our scientific examination of stretching. They might laugh at our serious discussions about when and how to stretch, and although they might be impressed with our scientific understanding of the body, they probably wouldn't be able to help but wonder, "Where's the spirit in it? Where's the heart, the soul?"

Probably one of the first formalized stretching programs was yoga, created in India more than two thousand years ago. Yogis used their practice to discipline their bodies, hone their intellects, and master their desires, so that they could "free themselves of delusions" and become one with God, who, they believed, was not an *outside* force but one who dwelled within. Yogis used the postures (or asanas) and breathing (or pranayama) as part of a devotional spiritual activity. Surrendering to the postures allowed them to clear the chatter from their minds and gather both physical and mental endurance so they could sit for hours in meditation. Yoga helped teach them how to maintain grace during discomfort (which made them better able to put up with life's little challenges in a positive frame of mind). This ability to change the perception of pain and turn it into pleasure was also an important spiritual aspect of yoga.

Around the second century A.D., a man named Patanjali wrote *The Yoga Sutras,* which was perhaps the first how-to book on stretching. But it wasn't so much about stretching the body as it was about stretching the mind. Patanjali outlined what he called the Eight-Fold Path of Enlightenment. Putting the body in various postures and quieting the mind were the initial steps toward reaching enlightenment. Some of Patanjali's other suggestions for obtaining enlightenment are still valid today:

- **Focus inwardly instead of on worldly distractions.**
- **Practice nonattachment to various outcomes.**
- **Turn off the senses.**
- **Meditate.**
- **Become aware of the oneness of all things.**

Regular practice of yoga is the first step on this path of inner peace. Many people who take up yoga today do it not only for health reasons but to find calmness and stillness in the middle of a hectic, modern world. Many other newcomers to yoga, however, simply embrace it as a formalized stretch class—and as a stretching exercise alone it can be quite valid (or quite extreme, depending on the style and teacher). Stretching isn't *always* the main point with yoga; there are internal forms of yoga that use no stretches at all. However, most forms of yoga not only deliver the health benefits of stretching but also stimulate or soothe the internal organs and endocrine glands, which regulate hormone production. (Thus yoga postures and many similar stretches can be especially good medicine for rebalancing women's hormone levels, especially during PMS, menstruation, pregnancy, and menopause.)

While yoga aims to unify the body, spirit, and mind, stretching is a more mechanical act, more "site specific." One could say, therefore, that yoga represents the sacred side of flexibility while stretching represents the secular. But since many stretches and yoga postures are identical from the outside, it's not so easy to tell them apart. One's internal experience is what really distinguishes stretching and yoga. You have the power to make regular stretching into a kind of yoga or simply to use yoga to increase your flexibility. As with all forms of movement (and many other things), you create the meaning in your mind.

Stretching as Mind-Body Medicine

The word "stress" comes from a Latin word that means "tight." When we try to cram too much information or activity into too little time or space, we get stressed. Our stresses come from both the inside and the outside. Outside stresses are to be expected and can be a good thing in moderation. Just as our muscles build strength against resistance, our minds may also expand and mature if we meet the outside stresses of life in a positive, open frame of mind. We run into health problems, however, if we let internal stresses pile up. Stress strains the nervous system and interrupts the normal functioning of the immune system, making us vulnerable to all sorts of stress-related illnesses, including high blood pressure and heart disease.

Breathing is one of the most effective ways to combat stress—and the effects are immediate. It acts like an instant tranquilizer, but unlike Prozac it has no side effects and doesn't lose strength the longer you use it.

Stretching is wonderful mind-body medicine, especially when combined with controlled breathing. As you move into a stretch, inhale through your nose. As you hold a stretch, exhale through your mouth. Try breathing down into your belly, especially in positions that allow you to do this comfortably. This not only lets you inhale "fresh" air and exhale the old but will allow you to enter into a progressively deeper and deeper form of total relaxation. Breathing alone is powerful medicine.

STRETCHING 101

CARE AND FEEDING OF YOUR STRETCHES

PHYSICIANS, PHYSICAL THERAPISTS, AND FITNESS PROFESSIONALS AROUND THE WORLD FOLLOW THE AMERICAN COLLEGE OF SPORTS MEDICINE (ACSM) RECOMMENDATIONS REGARDING CARDIOVASCULAR EXERCISE, STRENGTH TRAINING, AND STRETCHING. WE AT *FITNESS* FOLLOW THEIR GUIDELINES FOR STRETCHING AS WELL. THEY ARE THESE:

- Stretch the major muscle groups a minimum of two or three days a week, incorporating stretches into your overall fitness program in order to develop and maintain normal range of motion in the joints.
- Hold stretches for 10 to 30 seconds at the point of mild discomfort (the extra benefits you get from holding a stretch for 30 seconds to a minute are minimal).
- If you have time, repeat each stretch 4 times. According to ACSM's research, 4 repetitions (reps) induce the greatest gains in flexibility.

- For PNF stretching (tense-and-release stretching), hold the contraction for 6 seconds and hold the assisted stretch for 10 to 30 seconds.

If you're curious, the ACSM recommendations for other types of exercise are as follows:

- To develop and maintain cardiovascular fitness, take some form of aerobic exercise three to five days a week. Each session should involve 20 to 60 minutes of continuous activity; or you can try a minimum of three 10-minute bouts throughout the day at a heart rate of 55 percent to 65 percent of maximum for beginners (not so fit) and 65 percent to 85 percent of maximum heart rate for more advanced exercisers.
- To develop and maintain functional strength for muscles and bones, strength train two or three days a week. Do 1 to 3 sets of 8 to 10 exercises for the major muscle groups, reaching fatigue at 8 to 12 reps or 10 to 15 reps (using lighter weight) if you are a beginner.

More Nitty-Gritty How-to-Stretch Tips

Make each stretch a two-part event.

Think of the first 10 seconds as a prestretch. Gently stretch until you hit the first hint of tightness. Hold it there or back off from the stretch if it feels too tight. Spend the next 20 seconds stretching slightly further (even if just a millimeter).

Breathe.

Exhale as you stretch. If you're holding a stretch for 30 seconds, obviously it's hard to exhale the whole time. So inhale, then exhale and stretch; inhale, then exhale and stretch some more (repeat this as often as you feel necessary). The point is, you should coordinate your exhalations with the deepest parts of your stretches. Let your exhalations last longer than your inhalations. Deep breathing this way not only relaxes muscles but also lowers blood pressure and slows the heart rate.

When you "hit the wall," back off.

If, when you're stretching, your muscles start shaking, your neck curls, and your face grimaces in pain, you've gone too far. Back off from the tightness until you can *relax* in your stretched position.

Be relaxed before you stretch.

This may sound a little strange since you're stretching *to* relax. But starting off partially relaxed helps you improve your stretch. Do what you can to relax before you start. Breathe deeply. Visualize yourself in a relaxed state.

Use proper alignment.

None of the stretches in your stretch repertoire should force you out of safe neutral alignment or put any joints at risk. (All of the stretches we're presenting here are joint- and alignment-friendly.) Neutral alignment keeps your spine in a natural S curvature—a slight arch in the lower back, a slightly lifted chest, neck long, shoulders slightly down and pulled back, the abdominals and lower-back muscles in a slight contraction.

Some Frequently Asked Questions About Stretching

Should I stretch before or after workouts—or both?

You'll get the most lasting benefits if you stretch *after* your workouts, when your muscles are warm. But if you're like a lot of people, you might enjoy stretching before you work out. Is this a waste of time? Does it break a cosmic law? No. Many people like to take a moment to stretch before a workout, just to lengthen their muscles, "get into their bodies," and prepare their minds. There's nothing wrong with a preworkout stretch (in fact, many trainers and teachers still highly recommend it). But if you stretch before you work out, you should do it *after* a 5-minute warm-up. (Think of taffy. Hot taffy stretches. Cold taffy snaps.) If you insist on preworkout stretching, go for the mini 10-second stretch. Save your deeper stretches until the end.

What if I just want to get up and stretch. Do I have to warm up first?
No! Take mini stretch breaks as often as you like. Cats and dogs do it, and they don't warm up before they stretch. (They also don't hold stretches for a minute or bounce.) Try to stretch in the *opposite* direction from your "normal" bad posture. If you hunch over a computer all day, get up and arch your upper back. (Take your hands over your head and lift your chest to the ceiling. This stretches your shortened chest muscles and refreshes the discs in your upper back.)

I only have 5 minutes after my workout to stretch. How do I choose the best stretches?
Choose the muscles that you use most in your workout. For instance, if you run, you'll want to stretch your hamstrings, quads, and calves—not your wrists. If you're lifting weights for your upper body, you might want to stretch your lower back, abdominals, upper back, and chest. You might also work with a knowledgeable fitness trainer to evaluate which are your tightest muscles—and learn stretches to address those areas, in addition to strengthening exercises for your weakest muscles. (See our chapter on sports stretches for logical stretches to match your workouts and sports.)

Should I take a yoga or stretch class to increase my flexibility?
Yes, by all means! Formalized yoga and stretch classes with a qualified instructor *should* offer you the opportunity to stretch safely, learn proper alignment, and stretch muscles you might neglect on your own. But to increase your flexibility, you'll need to go two or three times a week. You can't expect to stretch one day a week and improve your flexibility. If you can only make the class once a

week, be sure to stretch on your own at least two other days a week.

My sculpting teacher wants me to hold a posture for 2 minutes. My whole body starts shaking when I do that. Is this wise?
No! As the ACSM points out, holding a stretch beyond 30 seconds adds minimal gains. This is not to say you can't hold stretches for a minute; just be aware that your most significant gains happen in the first 30 seconds. Yoga practice often involves holding a stretch for up to a minute, not so much for the flexibility gains, but to focus and train the mind. However, staying in a posture for 2 minutes or more can be counterproductive. At this point, the stabilizing muscles usually have to work very hard to keep you in the posture. This is hard work and increases your overall tension—during an activity designed to help you relax. In short:

- holding a stretch for 30 seconds is good for your muscles
- holding a stretch for a minute has minimal additional benefits for your muscles but may be good for your mind

I like to stretch every day. Is this too much?
That depends on how you stretch. If you stretch every day but do light 10- to 30-second stretches in a safe posture and with good alignment, the answer is no. As with most things, common sense rules. When tight, stretch, but don't overdo it.

I'm the tightest person in my stretch class. Should I be worried about this?
Stretching should be noncompetitive. There is no need to compare yourself to anyone else in the class—particularly if you are an "older body" stretching among younger females, who are naturally more flexible. Remember that your tightness is determined partly by genetics and partly by your behavior. If you're concerned about being tight, then get thee to a stretch class two or three days a week.

How do I know when I've stretched too far?

Pain! As we said earlier, forced stretching was used in medieval times as a form of torture. Believe us, you'll know when you've gone too far. The pain signals will start flashing inside you. Don't let that happen; stretch conservatively.

Are there "normal" ranges of flexibility, and how do I know where I fall in the scheme of things?

Yes, there is such a thing as "normal" when it comes to flexibility. Lie on the floor for a moment to take this test. On your back, put one foot on the floor, straighten the other leg, and lift it up in the air. Does the lifted leg make a 90-degree angle, perpendicular to the floor? That's normal. If your lifted leg is hovering close to your other knee, your hamstring is tight—you're less flexible than normal. You need to stretch. If your lifted leg hovers over your face (and you can pull it further), you're superflexible—more than normal.

Every joint has a range of motion. How little or how far you travel within that range determines your flexibility. Being able to travel through the whole range without pain or difficulty isn't always desirable. Being so flexible that other people cringe when they look at you may get you a job in Cirque du Soleil, but it can also dislocate your joints. (People like this are genetic rarities.) Traveling the middle path with flexibility is the wiser choice. We'll show you sensible (and also stiff and dangerous) ranges of motion for each exercise, later in this book.

Are there some stretches I should completely avoid?

This answer is different for everyone. There are not any absolute no-nos. A dubious stretch might help one person's athletic or dance performance yet put another person in traction. But there are indeed some stretches that make fitness professionals recoil in horror. Here are the "Seven Worst Stretches of All Time." If you're currently doing any of the following stretches, we advise you to reconsider safer alternatives. Although these may not hurt you now, they could later. Joint pain, after all, accumulates over a long period of time—and quietly. Warning signs come in the form of little twinges, creaks, and pains. But human nature being what it is, few people actually heed these warning signs until the problem has mushroomed into full-blown pain.

■ The hurdler's stretch

Sitting with one leg bent behind you and the other straight out in front, lean forward toward the straightened leg. This stretch commits a crime against the poor defenseless knee joint (already a fairly unstable joint; why pick on it?). This is supposed to stretch the hamstring. Actually, it is not a great hamstring stretch, and the forward flexion of the spine can overstretch spinal ligaments, especially if you round your spine forward and keep it unsupported (floating in the air). Bending the knee this way stretches the ligaments in the front of the knee, twists the kneecap out of alignment, and crushes the meniscus in the back of the knee. (Have you ever heard of a torn meniscus? It's your knee's worst nightmare. Join the Save the Meniscus Foundation!)

The hurdler's stretch alternative:

Sit up straight with your chest out. Extend one leg straight and bend the other knee so the foot touches the straight leg. Place one hand on your knee to support your spine and reach for your foot (or loop a towel or strap around your foot to assist the stretch), inclining your chest slightly forward, without rounding your back.

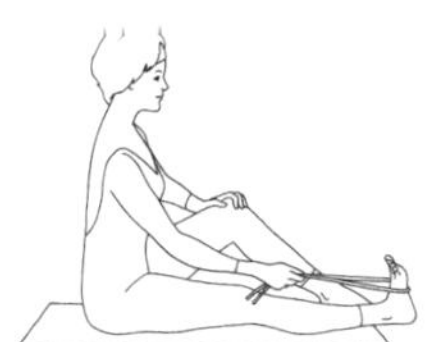

■ The hurdler's stretch, lying down

This stretch has started to reappear in some yoga classes. The idea is to stretch the quadriceps and hip flexors. Both knees are bent as you lie back. This stretch puts *both* knees at risk and can potentially damage the spine by putting extreme pressure on the vertebrae and discs. This posture also pinches nerves that run through the spinal cord.

The hurdler's stretch, lying down alternative:
To stretch the quadriceps and hip flexors, lie on your side. Bend your bottom knee for support (you can rest your head in your hand or lower your head onto your arm). Hold your top foot in your hand and pull the foot back, *away* from the buttocks. As you do this, press your hip *forward.* Avoid overarching your back. Use your abdominal muscles to stabilize and support your spine.

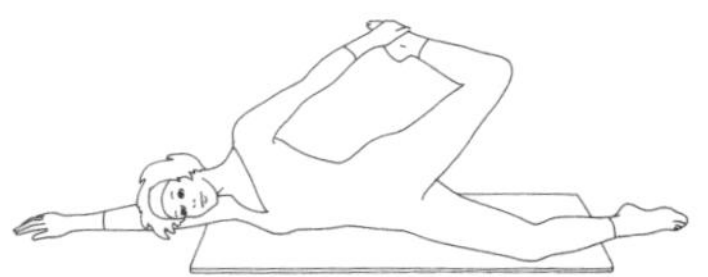

▪ The standing toe touch

Standing and touching your toes (with straight legs) used to be the "gold standard" for measuring flexibility. Fortunately, we've come a long way since then, although this supposed hamstring and lower back stretch can be found in yoga classes, with the spine both rounded and straight. Although some people may be able to do this movement without pain or discomfort, there are ways to make it safer, even for the very fit. (Whatever you do, don't bounce in this posture. That's one sure way to usher in the nasty old "stretch reflex.")

The standing toe touch alternative:
Take a wide stance, bend your knees, and place your hands on your thighs. Sit back into your heels to take the pressure off your knees and improve your balance. Start this stretch in a "squat position," with your back slightly arched, spine inclined approximately 45 degrees forward. Pull your

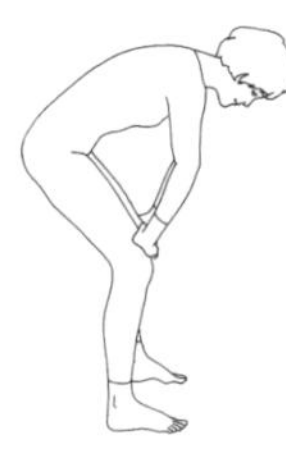

navel up to your spine as you round your lower back to stretch. You can do this a few times. Return the spine to the squat position and simply rise up as if coming out of a squat.

■ The unsupported back bend

There are many ways to assault your lower back in a back bend, whether balanced on your hands and feet like a gymnast, standing, kneeling, or lying on your belly. First, let's just say that arching your lower back *can* be a good thing, especially if you sit or slouch all day. But overdoing the arch, especially if you "sock it" to your lower back and let your abdominal muscles hang like jelly, is not. How far you arch depends on both the strength of your abdominal muscles and the health of your spine. This position, especially when taken to the extreme, can (just like the hurdler's stretch, lying down) compress the vertebrae and discs and pinch nerves running through the spinal cord.

The unsupported back bend alternative:

Try a moderate press up. Lie on your stomach, with your hands on the floor directly below your shoulders. Keep your abdominal muscles slightly contracted so they support the front of your torso like a girdle. Raise your head and chest off the floor. Avoid throwing your head backward (this compresses the vertebrae in your neck), but look up to the point where the ceiling meets the wall. This helps retain a forward head position without compressing the vertebrae in the neck.

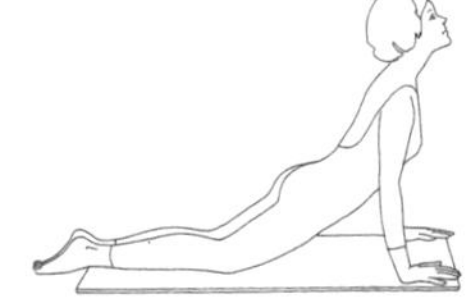

▪ The plow and the shoulder stand

The plow was banned from fitness classes in the 1980s (along with the standing toe touch). However, like some of the other banned postures, it sometimes appears in yoga classes. Granted, there are many versions of the plow, some less dangerous than others. The most dangerous versions hike your feet over your head, putting your center of gravity (most of your body weight) onto your neck. For one thing, this position takes a bad situation and makes it worse—most people's heads fall forward. Reading, working at a computer, watching TV with heads propped up on pillows all exacerbate a forward-head posture—and this gets worse as we age. (Stretching your chest and *gently* moving the head back or doing the moderate press up above [the unsupported back bend alternative] can help correct this.) But most importantly, the plow is dangerous because it can overstretch ligaments, it compresses the vertebrae in the neck and upper back, and it impairs breathing and blood flow. These same things can occur during a shoulder stand, where you lift your legs, hips, and back up perpendicular to the floor, supporting your entire weight on your shoulders and upper back.

The plow and the shoulder stand alternatives:

You can do the plow (to relax and stretch your lower and middle back) with your hands supporting your hips so the weight falls onto the lower—not the upper—back. This is a much safer version but not a very easy position to assume. To make a shoulder stand safer, maintain the same position as for the plow (with weight falling onto your lower back) and either lift your legs on an angle (with feet falling over your face) or straight up a vertical line. You can also

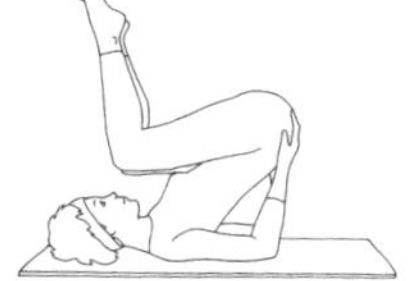

do these two plow alternatives with bent knees. The shoulder stand, done properly, can relax your lower back by changing your relationship to gravity. It also works your torso stabilizers.

■ The neck roll

It is a bad idea to roll your head in a full circle to stretch the neck. When the head is tilted back and to the side, the weight of the head shifts from the vertebrae into the small facet joints, which have little weight-bearing capacity. This can exacerbate a common misalignment of the neck vertebrae and compress the nerves that run through the spine.

The neck roll alternative:

Lie down with your knees bent and your feet on the floor. Lace your fingers together behind your head and lift your head off the floor so the top of your head curls toward your feet. Keep your shoulders on the floor or you will lose the value of this stretch. You'll feel this in your upper back as well as your neck.

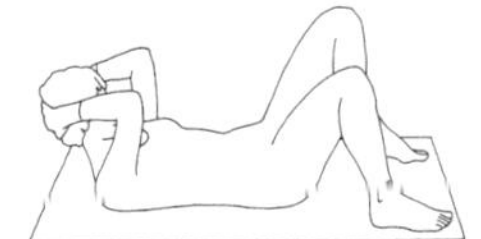

OURFAVORITESTRETCHES

LOWER-BACK STRETCHES

Lower-back pain is practically an epidemic in the United States, affecting 80 percent of the population at some point, and accounting for 25 percent of all workers' compensation complaints. A combination of sitting for long periods of time, poor lifting techniques, and bad postural habits all contribute to this. Backs "go out" both because of an imbalance between the strength and flexibility of torso and abdominal muscles and also because of tight hip flexors or hamstrings. To prevent lower-back pain, you need to do the following:

- Strengthen weak muscles.
- Stretch tight ones.
- Maintain good alignment and a vertical torso when you move.
- Avoid leaning forward without supporting the weight of your torso.
- Avoid excessively arching your spine.
- Be sure to use your legs when you lift heavy objects. Avoid rounding forward at the waist and creating a "banana back."

Even if you do all of the above diligently, lower-back pain may affect you anyway. When it does, your best bet is to move your pelvis gently ("wag" your tailbone side to side, forward and back, and/or in a circle). This warms and helps loosen muscles before you stretch.

1 HUG KNEES TO CHEST

Lie on your back and pull both knees up to your chest. Hold your arms *under* the knees, not over (that would put too much pressure on your knee joints). Slowly pull the knees toward your shoulders. This also stretches your buttocks muscles.

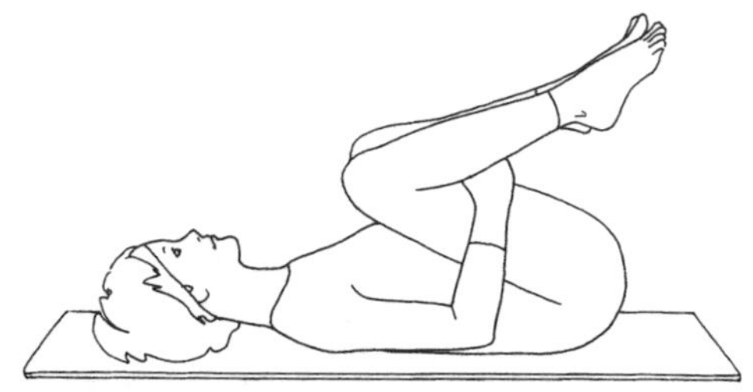

2 ERECTOR SPINAE STRETCH

This stretch lengthens the lower- *and* the middle-back muscles (the erectors run through the entire spine). Lying on your back, hug your knees to your chest, lift the soles of your feet toward the ceiling, grab your feet, and press your knees toward the floor. If you can't reach your feet, put your elbows inside your thighs and apply gentle pressure down. If you open your legs wide and place your elbows inside your knees, you'll also get an inner-thigh stretch.

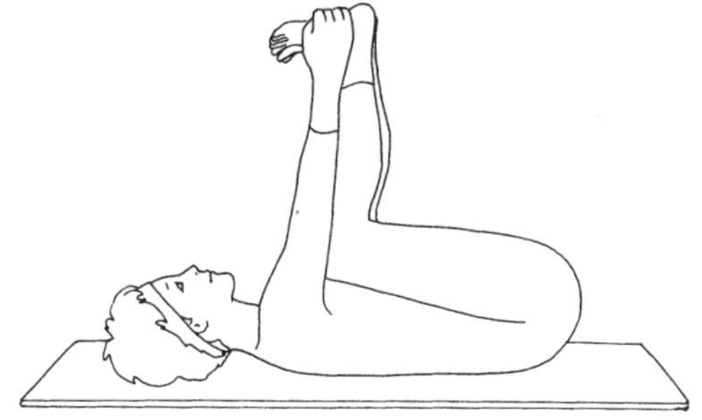

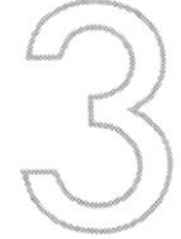

SEATED LOWER-BACK STRETCH

Sit in a chair or on a bench, feet flat on the floor, legs about hip-distance apart. Place your hands on your knees and slowly incline your body forward until your head and upper back hang forward between your legs. (To add an inner-thigh stretch, brace your elbows inside your knees and press your legs open.) Be sure to come up slowly so you don't get dizzy.

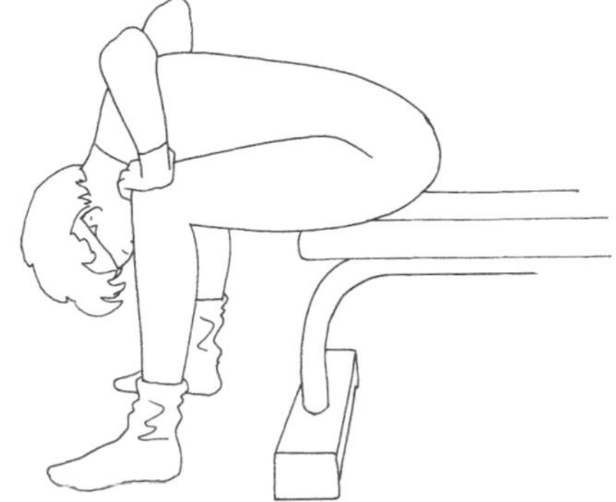

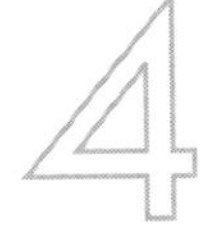

SEATED OR STANDING TWIST

Sit in a chair or on a bench with both feet flat on the floor. Rotate your head and chest to one side, so that at least one hand touches the back of your chair. Keep your feet planted. After you place yourself in this position, take a big breath and, on the exhalation, twist just a bit further. You can also do this standing about one foot in front of a wall (keep your back facing the wall). Place one or both hands on the wall behind you to stabilize your torso—and brace against your hands to twist your spine further. Switch sides.

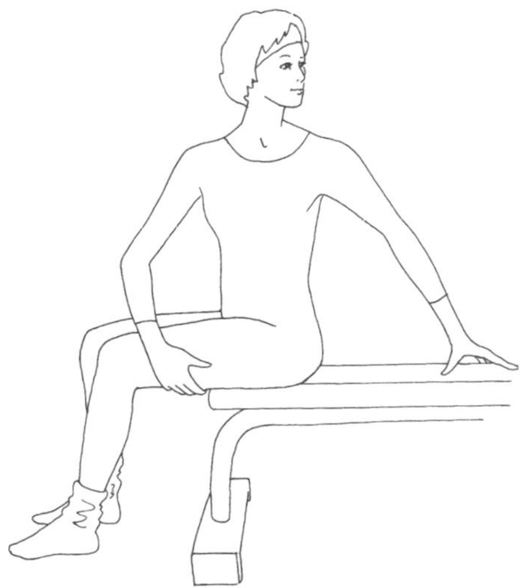

CAT STRETCH

On your hands and knees, pull your belly button up into your spine and round your spine completely—lower back, shoulders, and neck (let your head drop). Hold. This one's often paired with its companion—in which you gently arch your back. But it's the cat (the move with the humped back) that stretches the lower back.

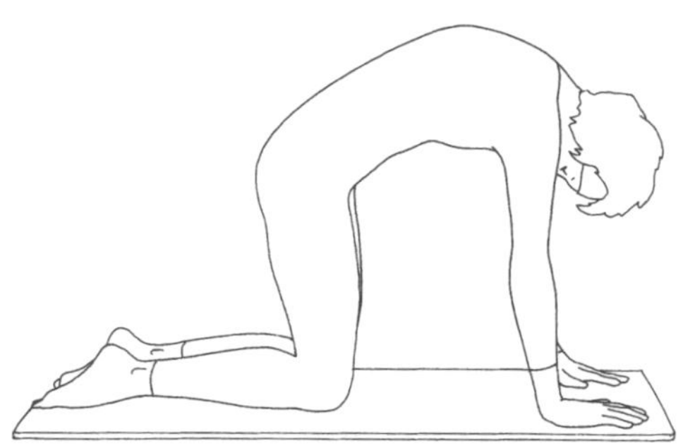

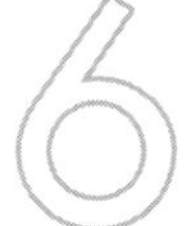

CHILD'S POSE

This works nicely right after the cat stretch. On your hands and knees, walk your hands in front of you. Lower your buttocks down to sit on your heels. Let your arms drag along the floor as you sit back to stretch your entire spine (pictured below). Once you settle onto your heels, bring your hands next to your feet and relax. "Breathe" into your back. Rest your forehead on the floor. Avoid this position if you have knee problems.

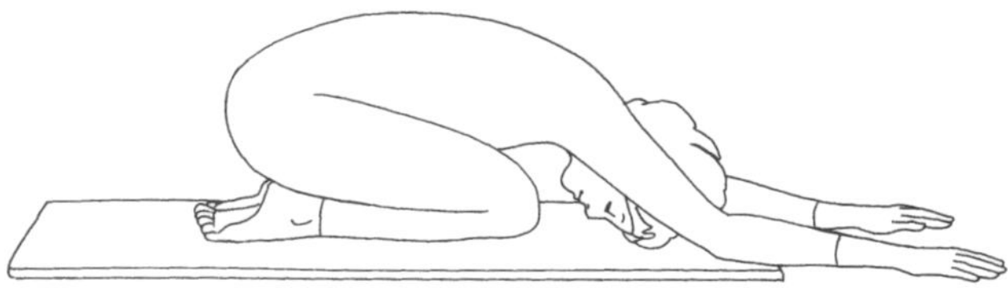

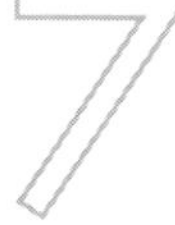

PELVIC TILT INTO BRIDGE

Lie down with your feet on the floor, heels directly under your knees, arms overhead to relax your upper back. Lift *only* your tailbone to the ceiling to stretch your lower back. (Don't lift the entire spine yet.) Pull in your stomach. To go into a bridge, lift the entire spine except the neck. The bridge isn't a lower-back stretch (it actually stretches the abdominals and hip flexors), but it is a mobility exercise for the lower back that relieves lower-back pain. This posture lets the fluid in the vertebrae trickle down to the *back* of the vertebrae (usually, in a slumped seated posture, that fluid falls forward into the discs). When you move into and out of the bridge, move slowly, one vertebra at a time.

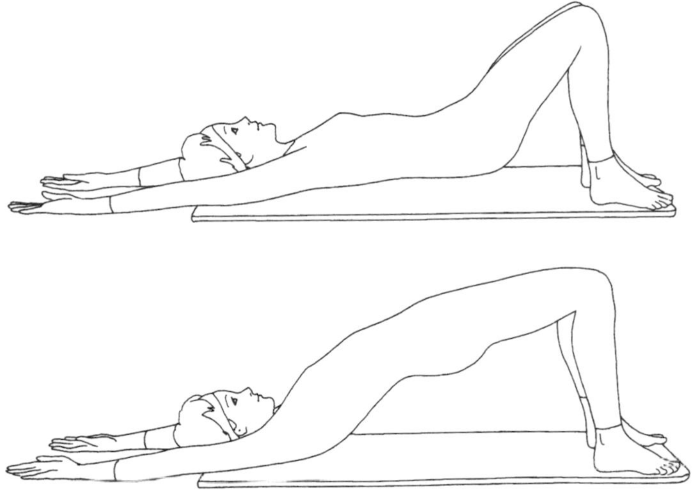

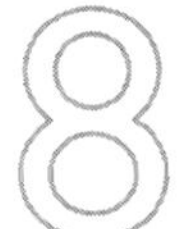

8 STANDING PELVIC TILT

Stand up with your feet hip-distance apart. Bend your knees slightly to keep them soft and "springy." You may want to move your pelvis forward and back a few times before holding the tailbone forward in this stretch.

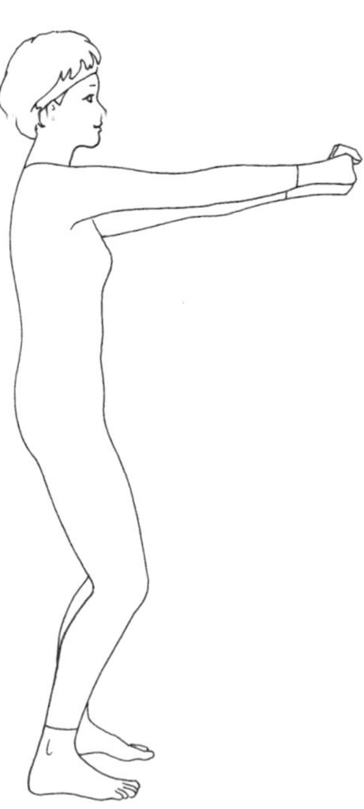

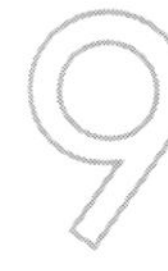

MORE ADVANCED STANDING PELVIC TILT

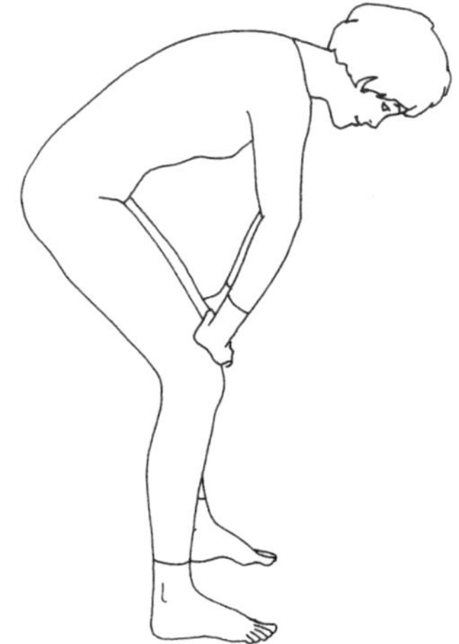

Take a wide stance, feet parallel and slightly wider than hips, with knees bent, the torso inclined forward 45 degrees and hands on knees (a squat position). Bring the tailbone forward to round the lower back. (This is also a good limbering exercise.) Round and arch the lower back a few times before holding the stretch. You can also deepen this stretch by involving the whole spine, from tailbone to shoulders. To stretch each side of your back, "drop" one shoulder to the opposite knee and hold. Avoid this position if your lower back feels strained.

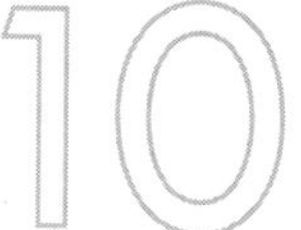

MODIFIED PLOW

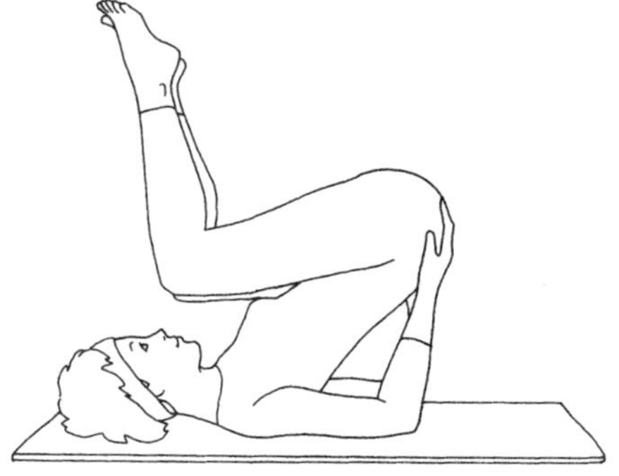

We don't like the old-fashioned yoga plow exercise because it compresses the vertebrae in the neck. This variation, however, is a challenging but very effective substitute. Lie on the ground and do the pelvic tilt into the bridge (stretch #7). Place your hands under your hipbones and keep your elbows on the floor. Lift one leg off the floor, then the other, and fold your knees toward your chest (feet can point up to the ceiling). This will shift your weight onto your lower back. Make sure to keep your center of gravity in your hips, not your shoulders.

11 THE FULL SQUAT

Avoid this one if you have bad knees. The full squat isn't as dangerous as you might think, however. In fact, it can be a very comfortable way to sit or work in your garden. (It's much safer for your back than bending forward at the waist.) The easiest way to get into a full squat is to hold on to an immovable object (a fixed pole or ballet barre, for instance). With a hip-distance stance, sit your hips back until your buttocks drop below your knees. Lower *slowly* to avoid knee trauma. (You can also try this with your back to a wall or without holding on to anything). Whatever position you choose, keep the weight on your heels, not on the balls of your feet. This also stretches your quads. Come up slowly.

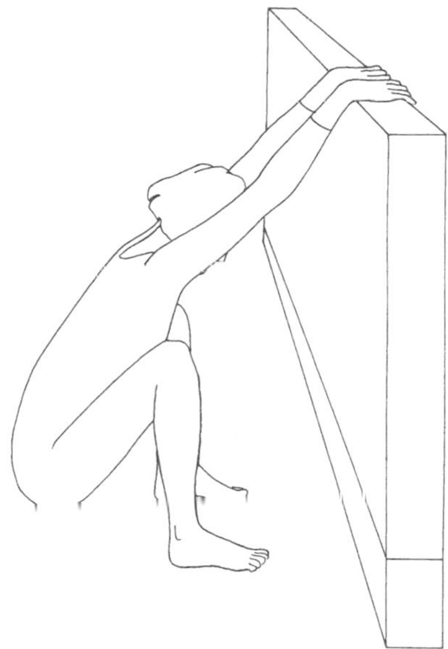

BUTTOCKS, HIPS, AND LOWER BACK

The gluteus maximus muscle is, as many of us realize, the biggest muscle in the body—but not the tightest. (That distinction goes to the jaw muscle!) Nonetheless, buttocks muscles need stretching too. You can tighten or pull a butt muscle when you run, skate, or walk, especially during the push-off part of the motion. Other buttocks muscles (the gluteus medius and gluteus minimus) rotate and lift the leg out to the side (called hip abduction). Smaller buttocks muscles also help rotate the leg in the hip socket. Tight buttocks muscles, therefore, limit motion in many ways.

Flexible and strong "turnout" muscles are especially useful for dancers. Dancers with good "turnout" can lift their legs higher and maintain greater control of all kicks, jumps, and leaps.

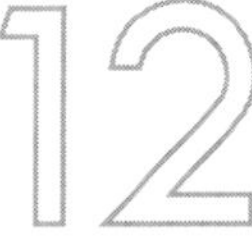

ONE KNEE TO CHEST

Lie on the floor with one leg straight and pull the other knee to your chest. Hold *under* the knee joint to protect the kneecap. Gently tug that knee toward your nose. Switch sides. This stretches the buttocks and lower back of the bent leg and the hip flexor of the straight leg. (For a deeper hip flexor stretch in this same position, see stretch #24.)

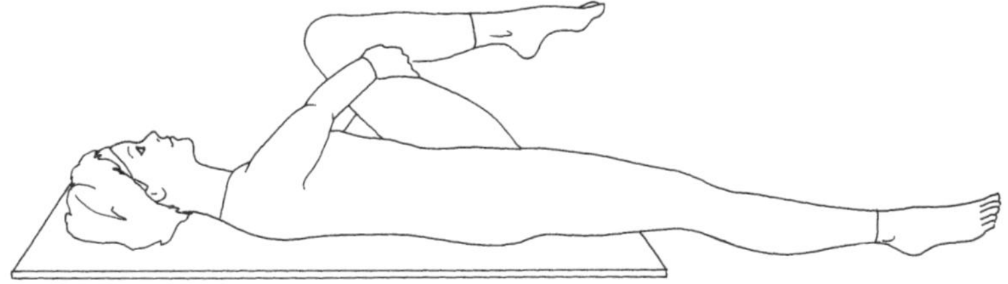

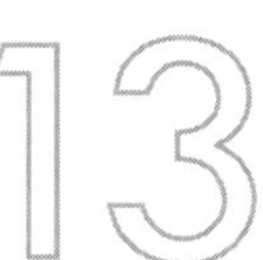

KNEE ACROSS THE BODY

Lie on the floor with your right leg straight. Bend your left leg and lower it across your body, holding the knee down toward the floor with your right hand. (The knee doesn't need to touch the floor if you're tight.) Place your left arm comfortably beside you and turn your head to the left. Imagine you have a weight tied to your tailbone. Let your tailbone fall back toward the floor as your chest reaches in the opposite direction to stretch your lower back. Switch sides. You can also do this stretch with both legs bent (easier) or with the knees crossed—as if sitting in a chair and crossing your legs (harder). Cross the left knee over the right when both knees fall to the right, and vice versa.

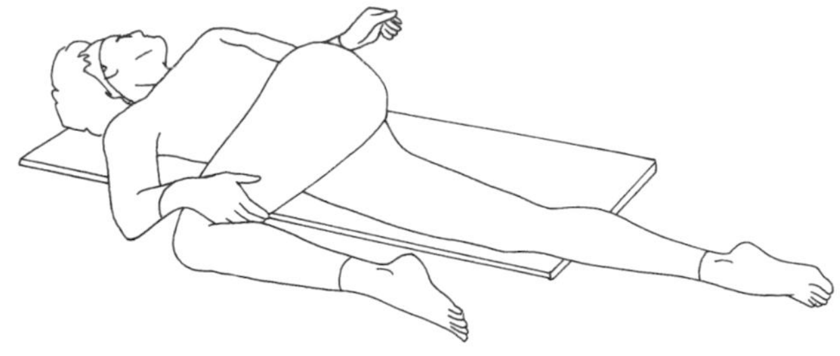

14 ANKLE ON THE KNEE

Place the right ankle on the left knee and pull both legs into the chest. Relax your neck and shoulders. Avoid the temptation to transfer your tension into the upper body. Switch sides.

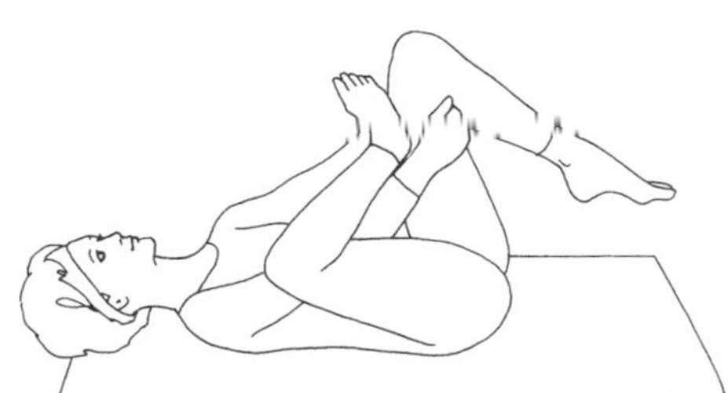

15 SEATED FLOOR TWIST

Sit up straight, balanced on your "sit bones." Keep your spine in neutral alignment (in other words, don't slump or excessively arch your back). Straighten your left leg, then cross your right leg over the left (put the right foot on the floor, outside the left knee). Turn your torso to the right, "hooking" the outside of your right knee with your left elbow. Put your right hand on the floor behind you for balance as you twist. Switch sides.

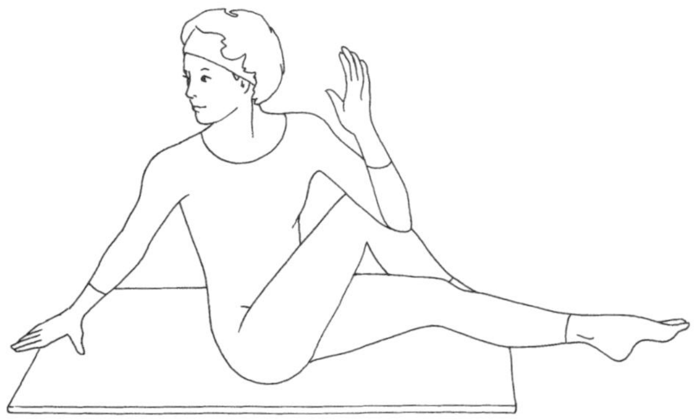

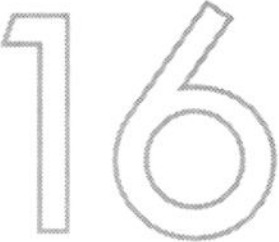

16

DANCER'S STRETCH

Sit up straight on your sit bones. Cross your right leg over your left, keeping the sole of the right foot on the floor and the right knee lifted up. Your left knee is straight and down on the floor. Place your right forearm on your right lower leg and your left hand on the floor. With a "flat back," incline your torso slightly forward and hold. The flat-back posture stretches the hip and buttocks. To stretch the lower back, slowly round the spine and let your head hang down. Switch sides.

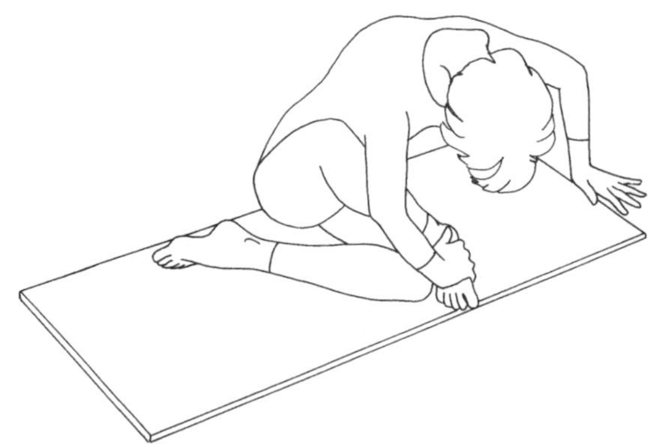

QUADS AND HIP FLEXORS

The front of the thighs (the quadriceps muscles, or "quads") take a lot of punishment when you run, walk up stairs, or squat down. Quads primarily help straighten (extend) your leg and lift (flex) your knee toward your chest. But the job of lifting your knee also goes to the hip flexors.

When you stretch your quads, you also have the option of stretching your hip flexors. A good rule of thumb is to focus on your quads first and make sure you can maintain good posture. Then, if you have the flexibility in your hip and the strength and stability in your torso to hold yourself in these positions, press the hip forward to stretch the hip flexor.

17 ON-YOUR-BACK QUAD STRETCH

Lie on a bench, table, or the edge of your bed and hang one leg and arm over the side. Bend the knee and hold the top of the foot. As you do this, be careful not to arch your lower back. Pull the belly button to the spine to stay in neutral. Press your foot *down* and into your hand (not up to your buttocks—which would stress the knee joint). To add the hip stretch, lift the hip of the leg you're holding up toward the ceiling. Switch sides.

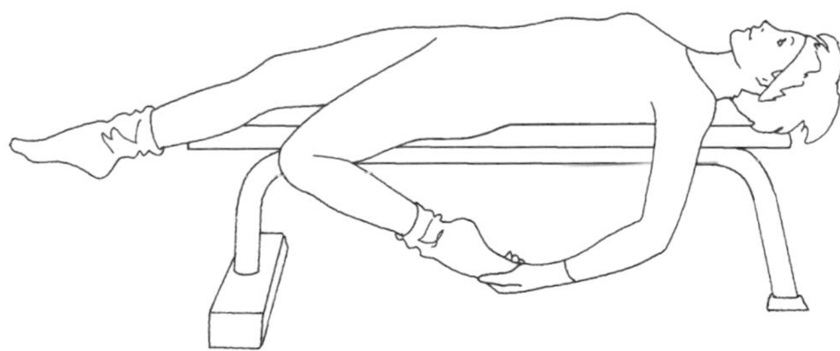

18

ON-YOUR-BELLY QUAD STRETCH

Lie facedown on a mat or rug with both legs straight. Bend your right knee so you can hold the foot in your right hand. Lift the foot up toward the *ceiling* (not to the buttocks) and raise the thigh a little off the floor. To stretch the hip flexor (if you have no lower-back pain), lift the thigh higher and press your abdominals into the floor to maintain torso stability. Keep your chin tucked under (you can rest it on your other hand) as you lift the leg. Switch sides.

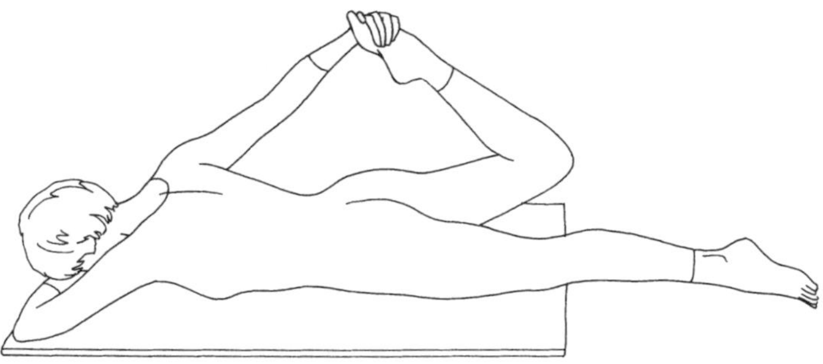

ON-YOUR-SIDE QUAD STRETCH

Lie on your right side, with your right knee bent at a 90-degree angle resting on the floor in front of you (this stabilizes the torso). Bend your left knee behind you and hold your left foot with your left hand. To stretch your hip flexor, press your left hip forward as you push your left foot *back* into your hand. Switch sides.

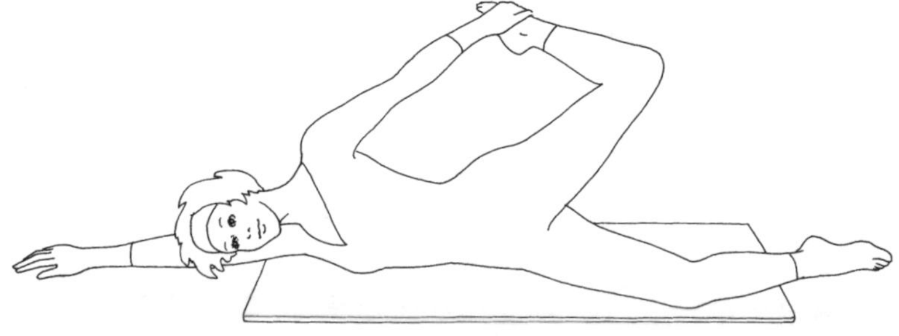

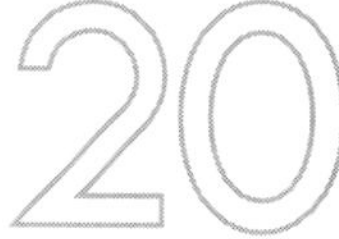

STANDING QUAD STRETCH

Stand on your left leg and pull your right foot up behind you with your right hand. To find and maintain your balance, soften your supporting knee (don't lock it or arch your back). You can also hold on to a wall, ballet barre, or pole if you need help with balance. Press the right foot *back* into your hand (not up to your buttocks). Keep your spine vertical throughout. Beware of tipping your torso and pelvis forward; that'll defeat the stretch. To add the hip flexor stretch, press your right hip forward. Switch sides.

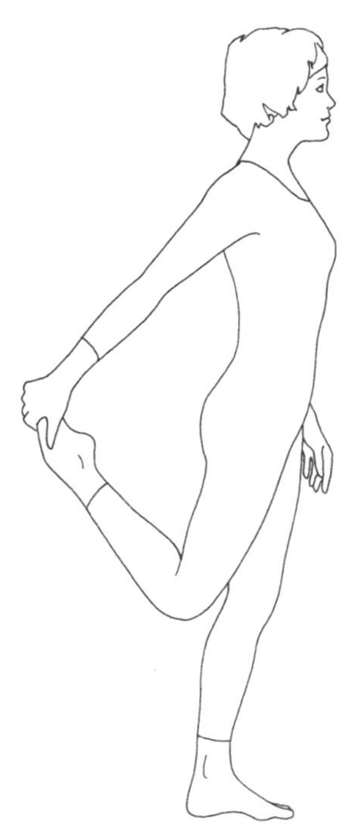

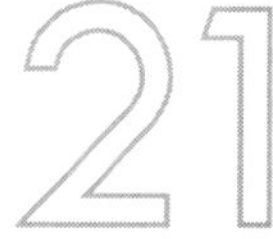

ALL-FOURS QUAD STRETCH

Balance on your hands and knees, then lift your right leg off the floor and hold the foot with your right hand. (Doing just this much works your torso and abdominal stabilizers.) Push the foot toward the ceiling (not the buttocks). To add the hip flexor stretch, press your right hip down toward the floor. Switch sides.

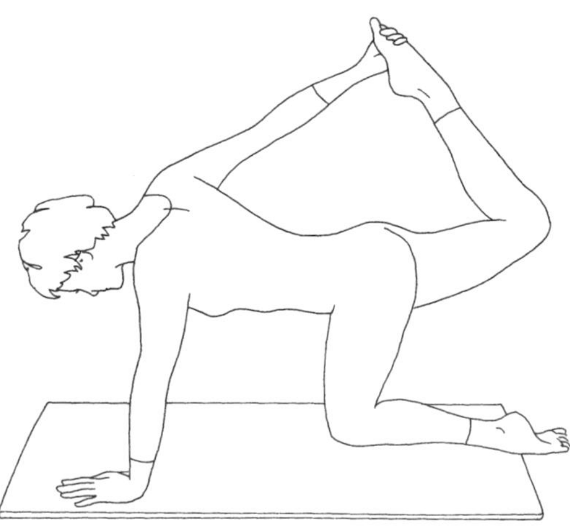

STANDING ELEVATED QUAD STRETCH

Stand with your back about two to three feet away from a bench or step. (How far away you stand depends on your leg length and how much stretch you want. The higher the bench and the further away you stand, the greater the stretch.) Lift one leg behind you and rest your foot on the step—either on your instep or the ball of your foot, whichever you find most comfortable. Keep your supporting knee slightly bent and avoid letting that knee extend out beyond your toes. Switch sides.

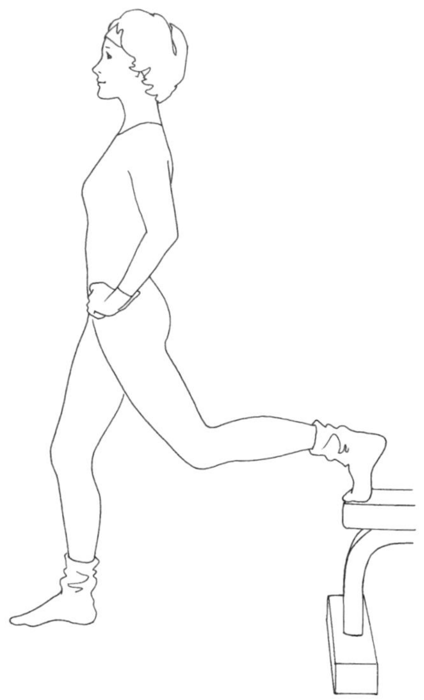

MOSTLY HIP FLEXORS

You can also stretch your hip flexors all by themselves if you keep your legs straight. Some bent-knee stretches (#26 and #27) also involve other muscles but put your focus on the hip flexors.

Hip flexors are very busy muscles. They lift the knees up toward the chest, provide a forward tilt of the pelvis (a pelvic tilt), and help rotate the thighs outward. When they get tight and short, they pull your pelvis forward and create a flat lower back, which can create a collapsed-looking posture.

Because hip flexors are naturally strong (and because one of the hip flexor muscles is located in the abdominal region), they can take over in abdominal exercises where both legs lift and lower to the floor. (That's why many of the best abdominal exercises immobilize the hip flexors.)

23 STANDING HIP FLEXOR

Stand up tall with the spine vertical, the left foot slightly in front of the right. Bend both knees and lift the back heel off the floor so you can press the right hip forward. You can't get a thorough, deep stretch in this position, however, because it's hard to relax the hip flexor and stand on it at the same time. Switch sides.

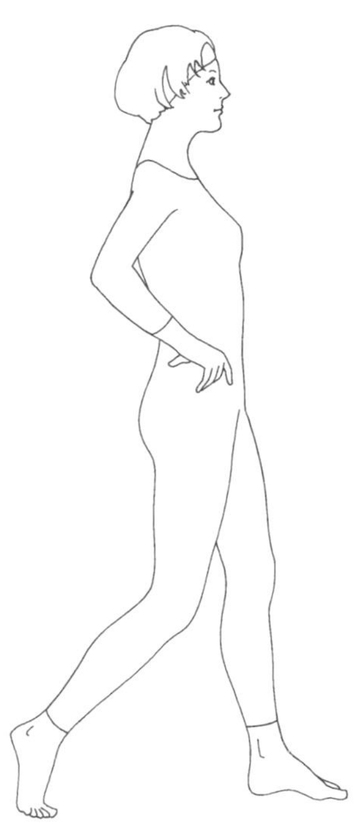

24 BENCH HIP FLEXOR STRETCH

Lie on a bench, table, or bed so that your buttocks are right up to the edge. Pull one knee to your chest and lower the other leg toward the floor (it doesn't have to touch the floor; it can hang in the air). Make sure you hold your spine in a neutral position as you do this (don't arch your back). Keep your lowered leg slightly bent for less stretch; straighten it for more. Switch sides.

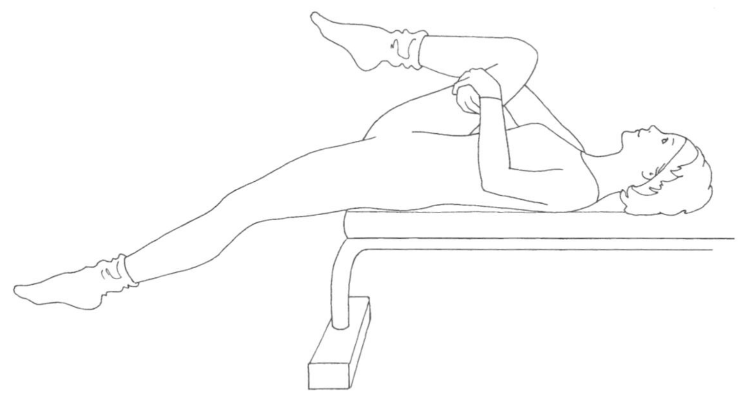

RUNNER'S STRETCH

It's easiest to get into this stretch if you start standing up, put one leg behind you, and slowly lower your torso down to the floor. Keep the front heel on the floor (if it lifts up, scoot your other leg further back). Place your hands on either side of your front leg. To get more out of this stretch, push your butt up toward the ceiling, and then gradually lower it back toward the floor. You'll stretch the hip flexor of the back leg and the hamstring and buttocks of the front. To make this easier, bend your back leg. To make it harder, straighten it. Switch sides.

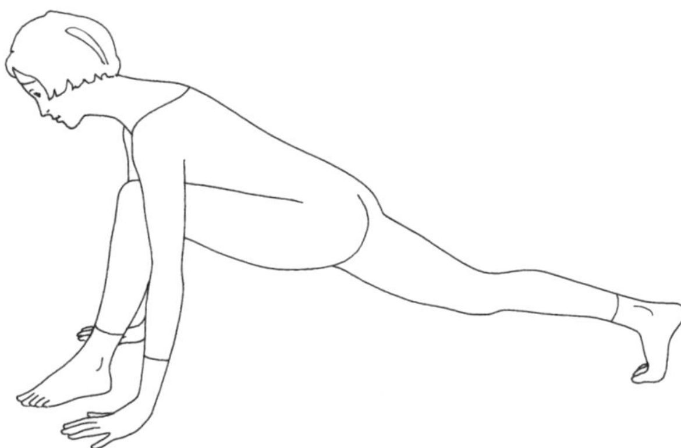

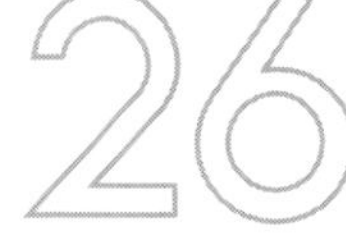

FOOT-ON-A-STEP STRETCH

Put your front foot on some sort of step or low wall about two to three feet high. Face the step head on and slowly bend your lifted knee. You can keep your spine vertical or inclined slightly forward. Be sure to keep your lifted knee over your ankle—don't let it shoot out over your toe as you bend the front knee. To maintain a healthy knee angle, press your weight into the heel, not the ball, of your foot. Although you'll certainly get a buttocks stretch here on your front, bent leg, concentrate on lengthening the hip of the back, *extended* leg. Switch sides.

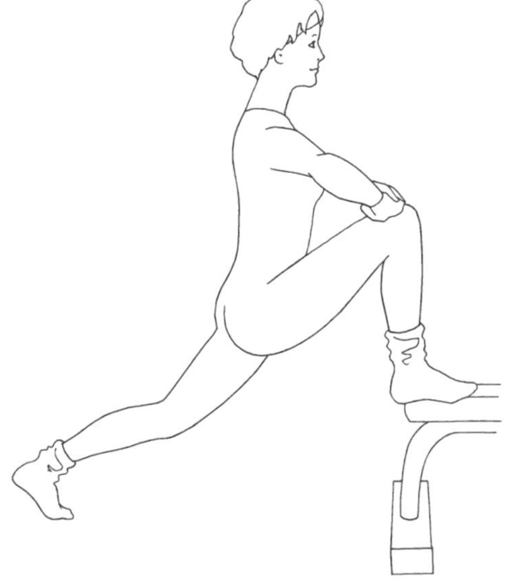

HAMSTRINGS

Tight hamstrings can lead to all kinds of problems. Short, tight hamstrings pull the spine into a swayback. They're also vulnerable to sudden moves. Hamstring pulls are so common because hamstring strength and flexibility tend to lag far behind that of their opposing muscle group, the quads. Whenever there's too much stress on the leg muscles, the weaker and tighter muscles tend to get hurt first. So it's usually the hamstrings or the groin muscles (the inner thigh) that suffer.

The hamstrings are also affected when the hip flexors (the front of the thigh at the top) are tight. Tight hip flexors put the hamstrings into a semipermanent stretch, which also predisposes them to injury.

The hamstrings cross two joints, the hip and the knee, and therefore are responsible for two motions: lifting the heels to the buttocks and extending the whole leg backward (as when you cross-country or telemark ski). Because of this, you can stretch your hamstrings in two ways:

- **with a straight leg (as in stretch #27).**
- **with the pelvis tipped forward and a "flat" back leaning out over the leg—which can be straight or slightly bent.**

Inclining the torso forward with a "flat" back is critical. (A "flat" back means your chest reaches forward and you maintain the slight natural arch in your lower back.) If you were to round your back forward as most people do (especially when trying to perform stretches #28, #29, and #30), you'd get a false sense of accomplishment. Rounding your spine lets your torso move forward, but that increases the flexibility in your lower back, not in your target here—the hamstrings. To stretch your hamstrings in stretches #28, #29, and #30, *don't* round your back.

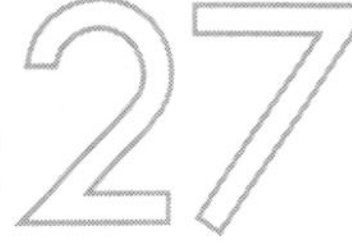

LEG-UP HAMSTRING STRETCH

Lie on your back, bend one knee, and put that foot flat on the floor to stabilize your spine. Extend the other leg in the air. If you're tight, you won't be able to straighten it. That's okay. Bend the knee so that the sole of the lifted foot faces the ceiling (or as close as you can get it). Slowly straighten the leg as much as possible and then pull the leg toward your nose. If holding your leg causes neck and shoulder tension, hold your leg or foot with a towel or strap instead. Switch sides.

Another way to do this stretch is to lie in an open doorway with your leg up the wall. Slowly scoot your body through the doorway until the wall supports the leg in an almost or completely vertical position.

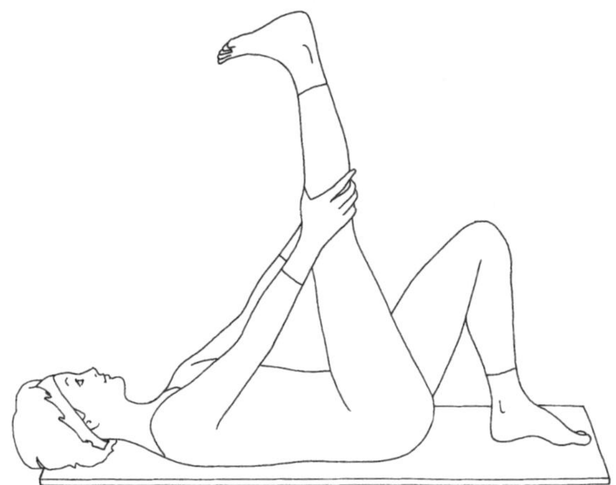

SEATED HAMSTRING STRETCH

Sit on the outer edge of a chair or bench and put one foot on the floor (the knee should be bent at a 90-degree angle). Extend your other leg in front of you (slightly bent or straight) with the toes flexed toward the ceiling. Place your hands on the thigh of your bent leg and incline forward with a "flat" back. Switch sides.

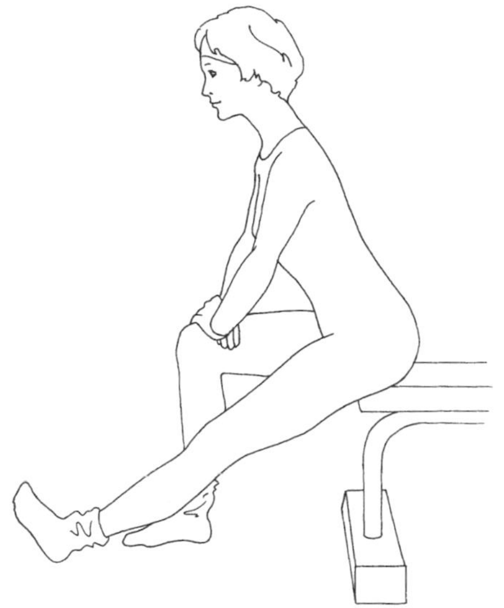

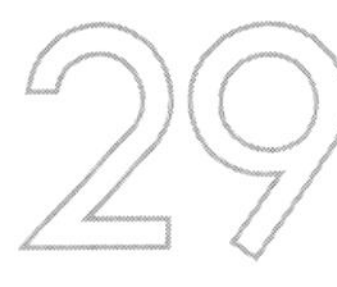

FLOOR OR BENCH HAMSTRING STRETCH

To do this on the floor, sit up straight and bend one leg so that the foot touches the floor. Straighten the other leg as much as possible and flex the toes up. With a "flat" back, incline your torso forward. Think of sending your hips back as you do this. Place one hand on your knee to support your spine and reach for your foot (or loop a towel or strap around your foot to assist the stretch).

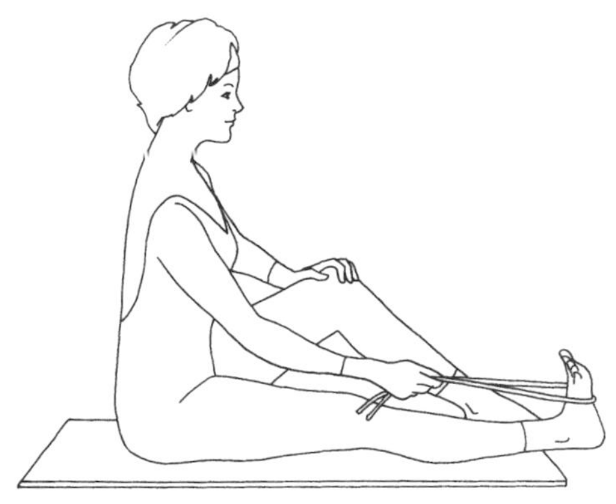

To do this same stretch sitting on a bench or low wall, simply sit with your straight leg on the bench and the other foot on the floor. Stretch as above. Switch sides.

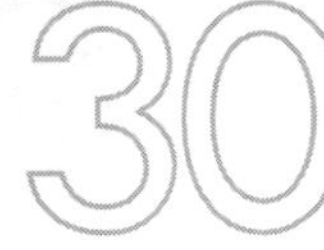

STANDING HAMSTRING STRETCH

You can do this with your foot on the ground or elevated on a wall. Stand up straight and extend one leg in front of you (slightly bent or straight) with your foot flexed. Bend your supporting knee and incline your torso forward, again with a "flat" back. Place your hands on your thighs—not on your knees (you might inadvertently press down on the knee joint). Switch sides.

For a deeper stretch, elevate the leg being stretched on a bench, step, or wall.

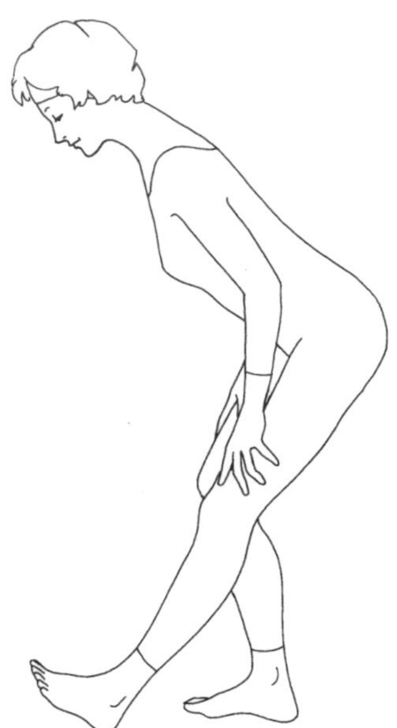

OUTER HIP AND THIGH

The outer hip and thigh muscles sometimes get attention during buttocks and lower-body stretches (see stretches #11–#16). However, these muscles (the gluteus medius, gluteus minimus, and tensor fasciae latae, collectively called the abductors) occasionally beg for your undivided attention. Because abductors help you step side to side and rotate your leg in and out in the hip socket, tight abductors can cause pain or unsteadiness when you walk. These muscles aren't easy to isolate and stretch alone, however. To do so, you have to get creative.

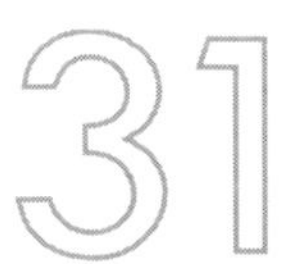

SIDE-LYING FLOOR STRETCH

Lie on your left side, bending your left knee in front of you to stabilize your torso (use your abdominal muscles as well to hold you upright). Straighten your right leg and rest the right foot on the floor *behind* your left. Straighten your right arm over your head and gently pull on your right wrist to stretch the entire right side of the body. Switch sides.

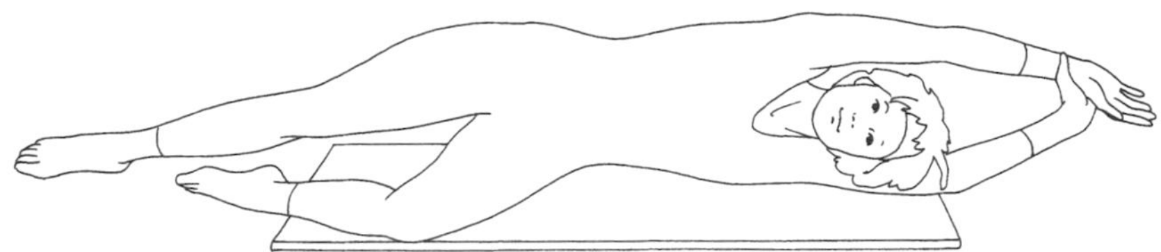

32 SIDE-LYING STRETCH ON A BENCH

Prop yourself on your left side on a bench, aerobic step, table, or bed. Extend your left arm out, and rest your head on it. Adjust your body so the right leg can drape off the end. (Leave yourself enough bench in *front* of your left supporting leg so it has a place to rest.) If your bench is too high, you can rest the right foot on a block or chair that's slightly lower than your bench. Be careful not to let the leg hang down at too drastic an angle, especially if it's very tight or if this causes you any pain in your lower back. Switch sides.

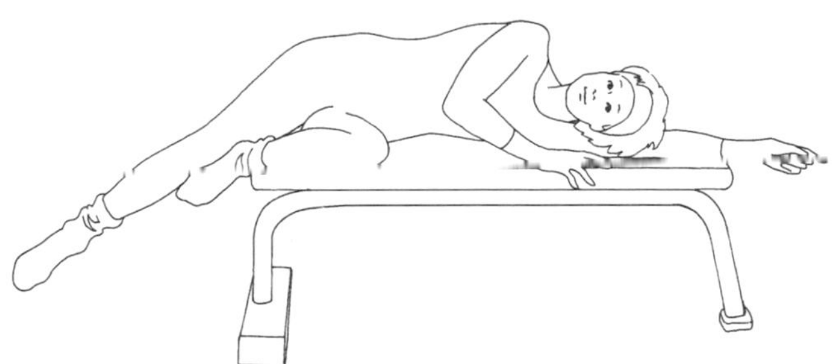

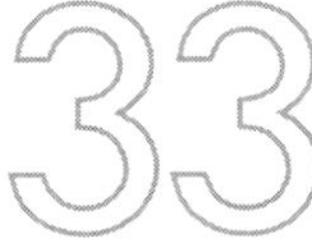

33 STANDING SIDE HIP STRETCH

Stand with your feet shoulder width apart and shift your weight onto your right leg. Bend your right knee and "sink" your weight down into that leg. Let the right hip push out to the right. To deepen the stretch, extend your left arm overhead, toward the left. Switch sides.

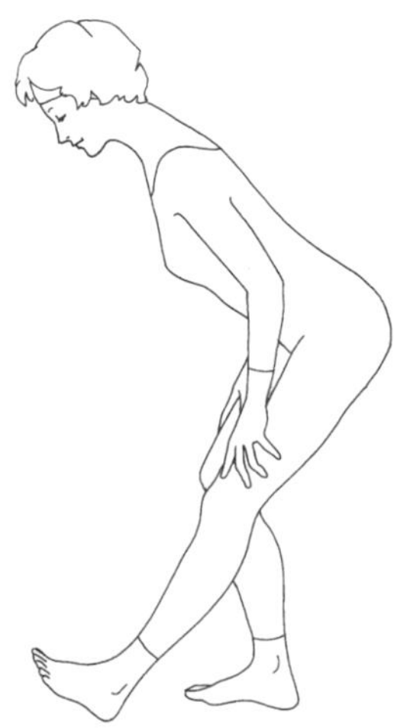

INNER THIGH

The inner-thigh muscles (or adductors) help you cross your legs over the center line of your body, rotate your legs in the hip sockets, and flex your knees. Like the hamstrings, they're vulnerable to injury. But stretching and strengthening them can prevent problems.

To stretch your inner thighs, you need to use straddle positions (standing, seated, and so on) with your legs either bent or straight. You don't need a perfect 180-degree extension to have good, functional inner-thigh mobility. A little inner-thigh stretching goes a long way.

34 SEATED BUTTERFLY STRETCH

Sit up straight, balancing on your sit bones. Touch the soles of your feet together with your feet six to eight inches in front of your hips. (Don't pull your feet in too close—that's tough on the knees.) Rest your elbows or hands on your inner thighs (relax your shoulders as you do this) and incline your chest forward. You don't need to round your shoulders to perform this stretch.

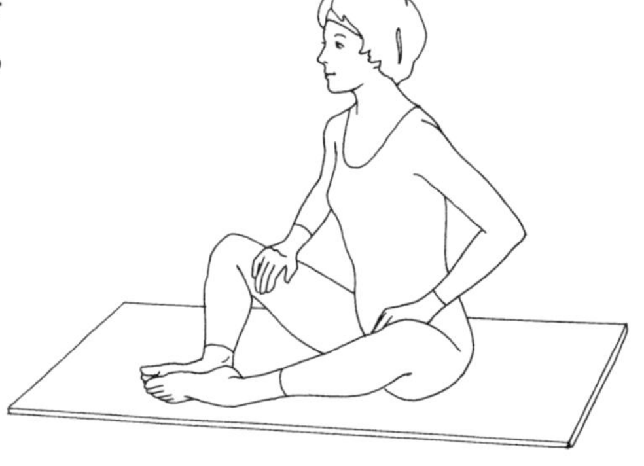

35 SIDE-LYING GROIN STRETCH

Lie on your right side and bend your right knee in front of you to stabilize the torso. Rest your head on your right hand or shoulder. Lift your left leg upward and hold it by the back of the knee (easier) or the foot (harder). Pull your left knee in toward your left shoulder and simultaneously press your foot or knee down to the floor. To intensify this stretch, straighten your left leg. Switch sides.

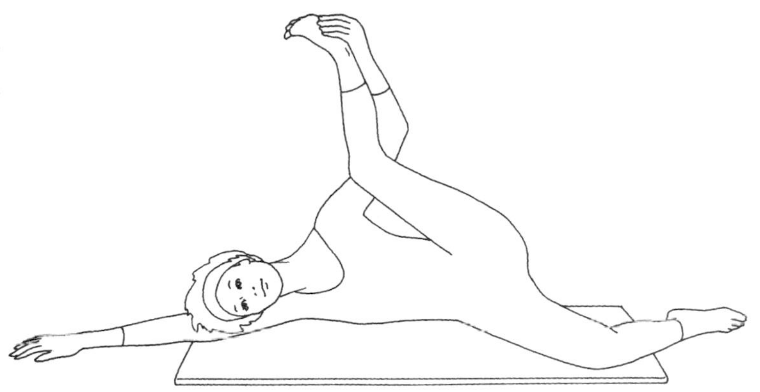

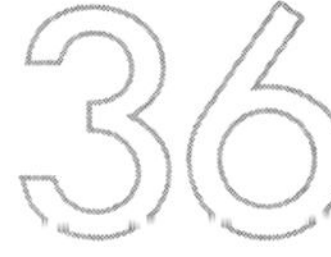

36 HANG OVER A CHAIR

Standing next to a chair or bench, put your left foot up on the chair or bench. Position your legs in a straddle, about 1½ times the width of your hips. Bend your right knee and lean your torso forward over your legs and hold. Avoid rounding your spine. Place your hands on your thighs for support. Switch sides.

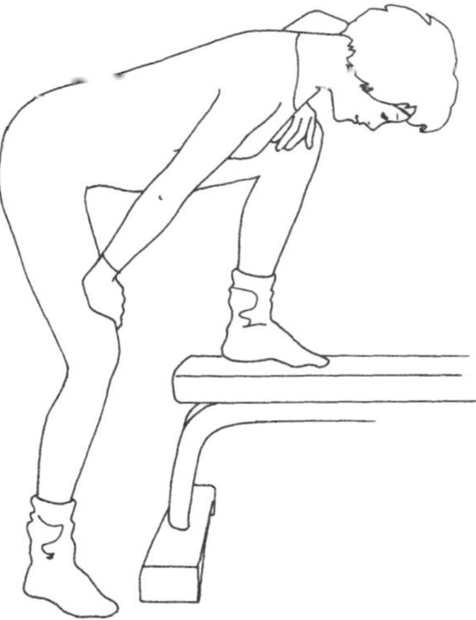

STANDING INNER-THIGH STRETCH

Prop your left foot on a bench, chair, fence, or ballet barre and straighten that leg so it's directly to your side or slightly forward. (The higher your leg, the harder this is. Work within your limits.) Your supporting leg should be far enough away from the bench so that you can stand comfortably and your knee won't jut out over your toes. Bend your right knee so that your hips drop slightly. To add a torso stretch, place your left hand on your hip for support and lift your right arm overhead to the left. Switch sides.

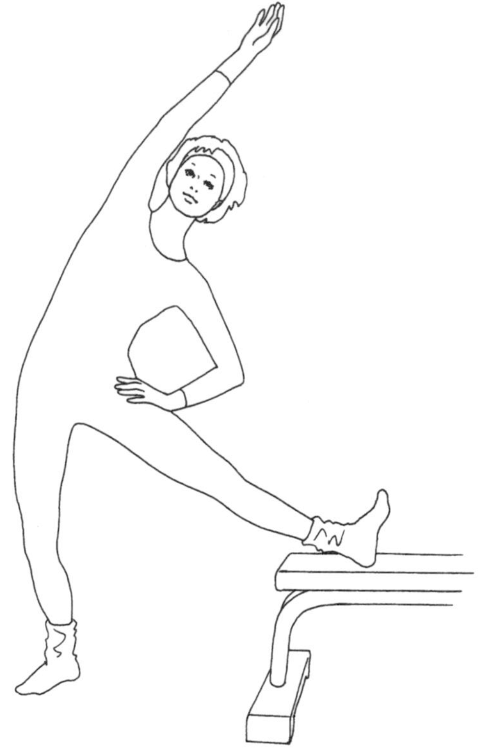

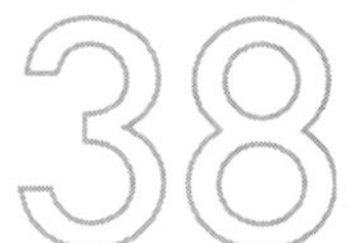

THE STRADDLE

There are many variations on straddles. Whichever one you choose, begin in a seated, upright position, balancing on your sit bones. (If you can't balance without rounding your back, you're not ready for this stretch.) Start by extending your legs in front of you in a V. To make this easier, bend both knees so that both feet touch the floor. To make it harder, straighten both legs. Whichever position you choose, keep your back straight with your hands on the floor in front of you as you incline your torso forward—and keep your neck long and in line with your spine.

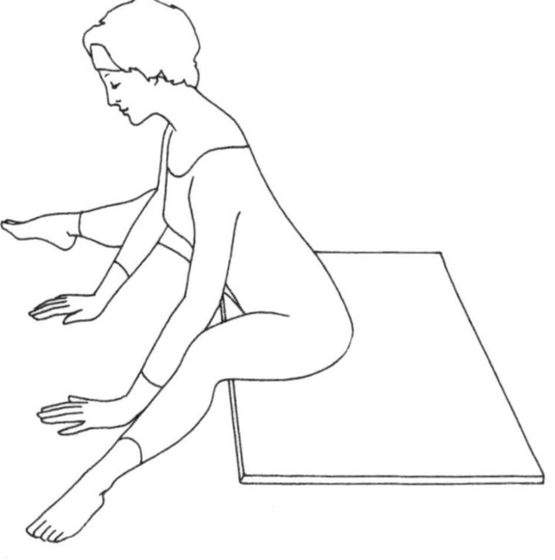

CALVES AND ACHILLES TENDON

Calves were designed for endurance. If they fatigued too easily you wouldn't be able to walk all day without doubling over from lactic acid burn. But just because they're tough doesn't mean they don't need stretching. Tight calves make you prone to injury. Any time you go for a run without warming up and stretching your calves, run on the balls of your feet (which tightens the calves), run on hard surfaces, make a sudden wrong move, or train when you're fatigued (many calf pulls come at the end of a workout), you're at risk for injury.

Your two main calf muscles (the gastrocnemius and the soleus) both help you point and flex your feet. To stretch the "gastroc," keep the leg straight. To stretch the soleus, bend the knee slightly (you can turn stretches #39, #40, #41, and #43 into soleus stretches by slightly bending the knee). Soleus stretches also stretch the Achilles.

At their lower ends, the gastroc and soleus both attach to one tendon, called the Achilles. Although this is the largest and strongest tendon in the body, it's not immune to injury. Women who wear high heels are most prone to Achilles injuries because having the heels chronically elevated shortens the Achilles tendon. Although it's a tendon and therefore not very flexible, it needs some stretching too. Stretch your Achilles after your calves.

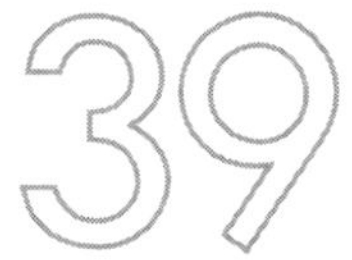

STANDING CALF STRETCH

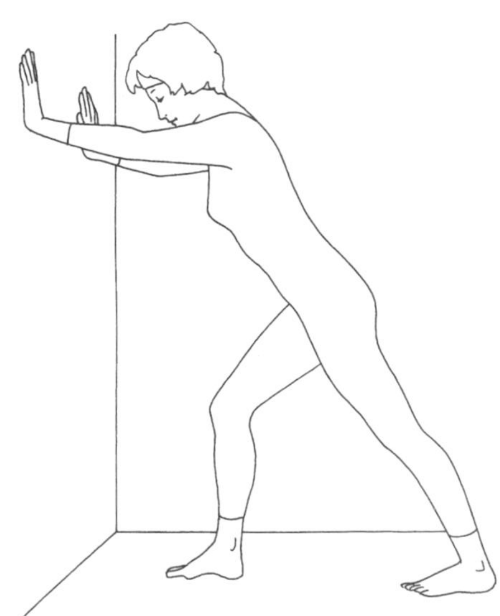

Face a wall or a fence and put both hands on the surface in front of you. Extend one leg straight behind you. Bend the other leg so that the knee doesn't extend over the toes. Incline your torso forward, keeping the extended heel down. Ideally, you should try to maintain a straight, diagonal line from the heel to the top of your head. To add a soleus and Achilles tendon stretch, bend your

back knee but try to keep the heel on the ground. Be gentle with it. Never force a tendon stretch. Switch sides.

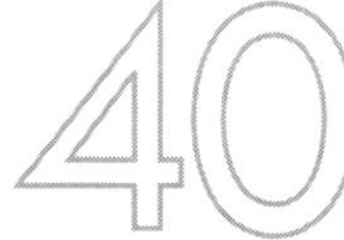

SUPINE CALF STRETCH

Lie on your back and put one foot on the floor to stabilize your torso. Lift the other leg in the air and using a belt, towel, or your hand if you can reach, gently pull the toes down to the floor without hyperextending the back of the knee. Switch sides.

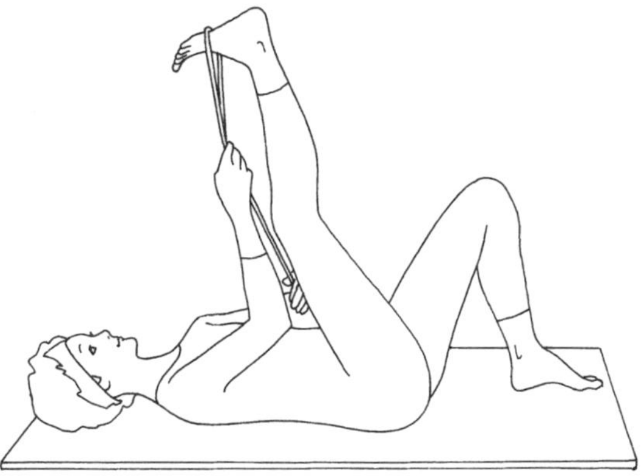

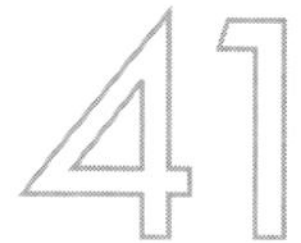

SEATED CALF STRETCH

Sit up straight, balancing on your sit bones. You can also do this with your back against a wall for more back support. Bend one knee and put that foot on the floor to stabilize the torso. Straighten your other leg and flex your toes to the ceiling. Using a belt, towel, or your hand if you can reach, pull the toes toward you with your back flat. Make sure you don't compromise your spine to do this; keep your back straight, not rounded. Switch sides.

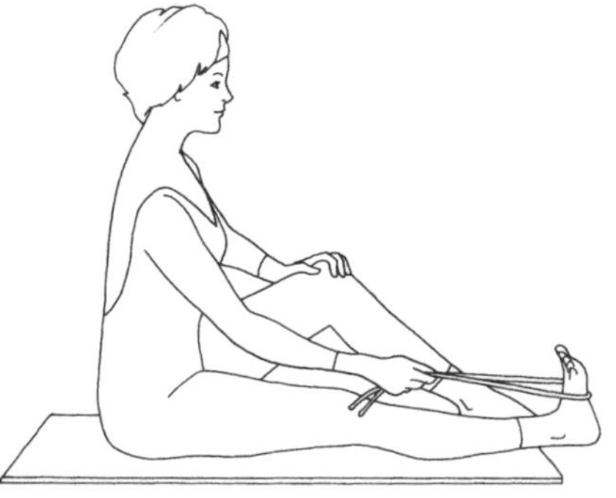

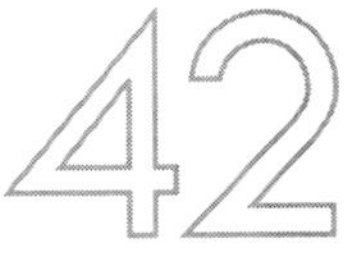

42 STANDING SOLEUS AND ACHILLES STRETCH

Stand with your feet hip-distance apart, one foot slightly in front of the other. Bend both knees, keeping your back heel on the floor. Switch sides.

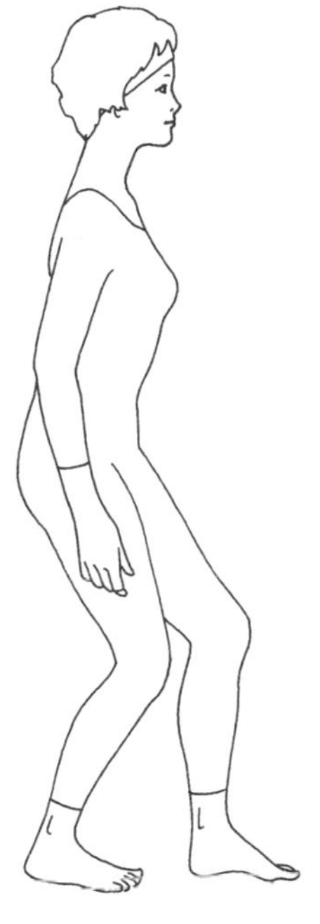

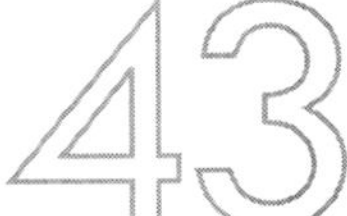

43 THE STAIR STRETCH

This stretch gives you the fullest range of motion for your efforts, but you might not be ready for this full stretch if your calves are very tight. Stand on a stair with one heel over the edge (keep your other foot on the step and bent slightly). Gently lower the heel as much as you can. Switch sides.

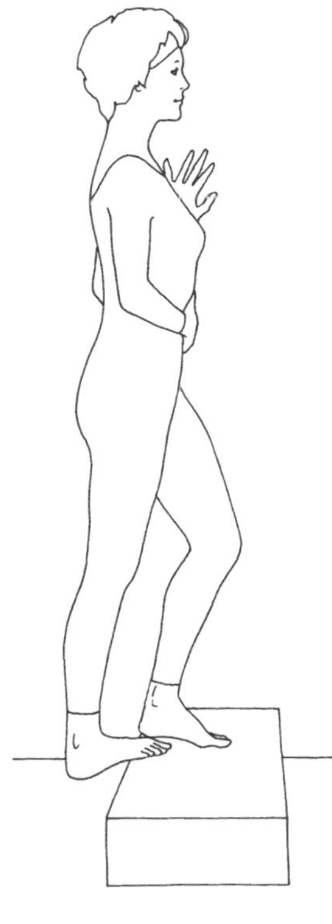

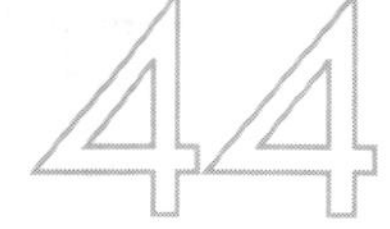

STARTING-BLOCK ACHILLES STRETCH

Crouch down with one knee forward, the other foot tucked underneath you as if in a runner's starting block. You don't need to sit on that back foot—spare your knee! Lean your torso forward onto your front thigh. That will lift your front heel slightly off the ground. Switch sides.

ABDOMINALS

It's easy to forget about stretching the abdominals. Most of us have to force ourselves to contract them with exercise. Still, the abdominals, like all muscles, need to be lengthened, especially since they spend much of their waking hours in a shortened, slumped position. Stretching the abdominal muscles also offers relief to the spinal vertebrae.

The trick to stretching the abdominals effectively is not to arch the spine too much. A *slightly* extended, as opposed to an overly extended, spine is all you need. This motion is a normal part of life. In fact, most physical therapies for the spine include a certain degree of controlled flexion. However, if you suffer from a weak or painful lower back, be especially cautious when arching your back. Avoid any range of motion that causes sharp pain, and make sure you're warm before you stretch.

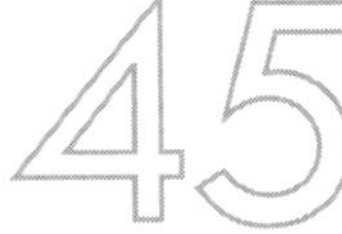

FULL-BODY STRETCH

Lie on your back with your arms overhead. Raise your chest to the ceiling and let your lower back lift off the floor. Suck in your belly button toward your back and reach your arms and legs in opposite directions.

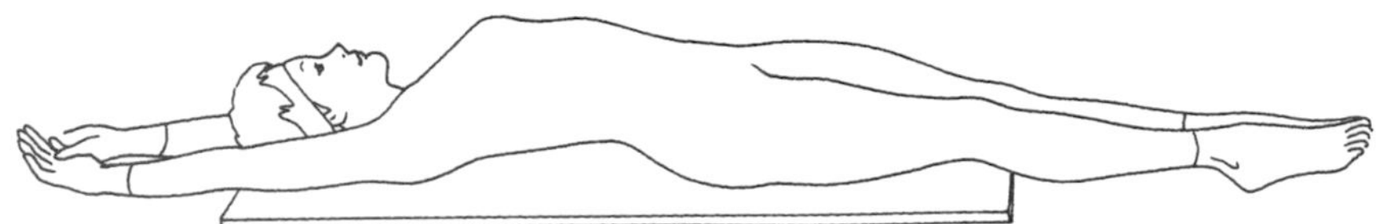

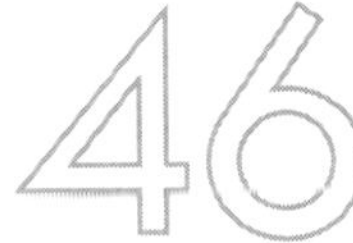

UPWARD-FACING DOG

Lie facedown and place your hands on the floor just outside your shoulders. To start, rest on bent elbows and forearms. Only progress once you're flexible enough. Press into your hands to lift your head, shoulders, upper body, and hips off the floor. You should be balanced on your hands and thighs. Keeping the hips down on the floor will cause too extreme an arch in your lower spine. To minimize strain in your shoulders, make sure your arms hang straight down from the shoulders, perpendicular to the floor.

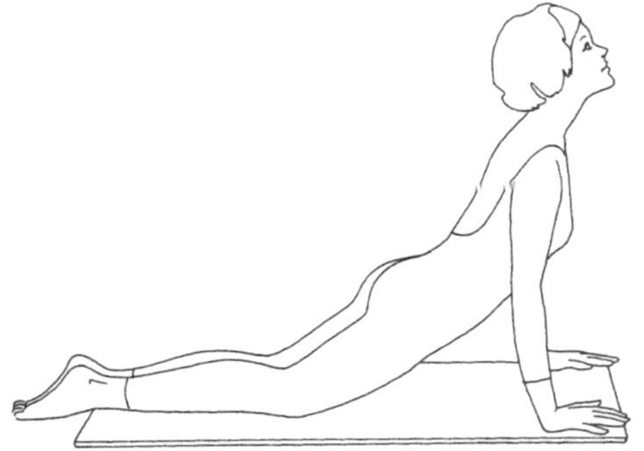

47 ONE-HALF LOCUST

Lie facedown on the floor. Put your left hand under your left hipbone to pad your hip and pubic bone. Bend your right knee so you can hold the foot in your right hand (this begins just like stretch #18 for quads). Lift the foot in the air and simultaneously lift your shoulders off the floor. This also stretches the right hip flexor and the chest and shoulders. Switch sides. If this doesn't bother your back, you can try it with both arms and legs at the same time.

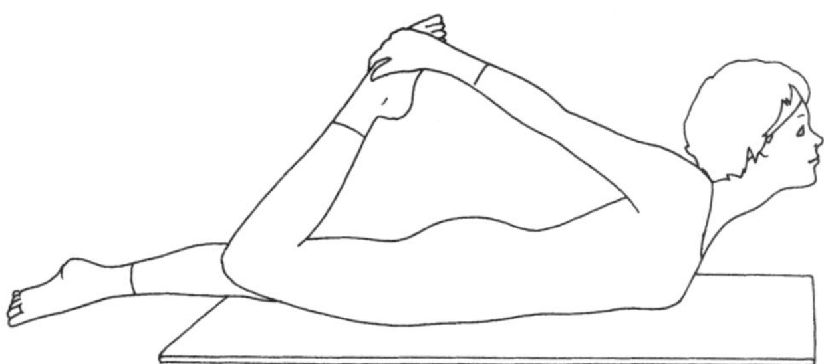

OBLIQUES AND TORSO

Torso stretches can involve many muscles: lats (latissimus dorsi), erectors, abdominals, obliques, pectorals, and others. Since we address many of those specific muscles elsewhere, think of these torso stretches as general trunk stretches, with a little additional shoulder stretching.

Pay close attention to the form in the lateral stretches (ones that go to the side) since, despite their popularity, these stretches tend to be poorly executed. Take each lateral stretch one step at a time.

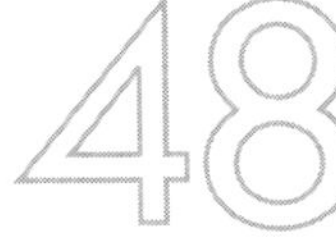

OVERHEAD STRETCH

Standing, lace your fingers together and open your palms to the ceiling. Keep your shoulders down as you extend your arms up. To create a full torso stretch, pull your tailbone down and stabilize your torso as you do this. Stretch the muscles on both the front and the back of the torso.

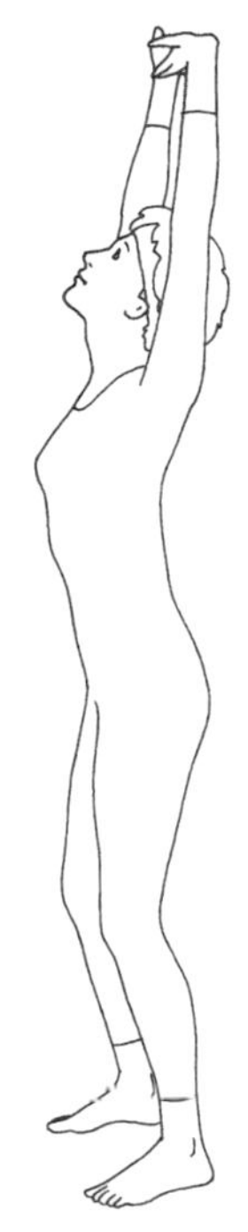

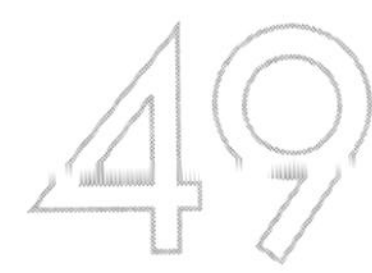

STANDING LATERAL STRETCH

Take a slightly wider than hip-distance stance with your knees slightly bent. Place your right hand on your right hip to support the spine. Raise your left arm in a vertical line and place your left hand behind your head. Keep it there as you incline your torso to the right. Keep your weight equally distributed between both legs (don't lean into your left hip). Switch sides.

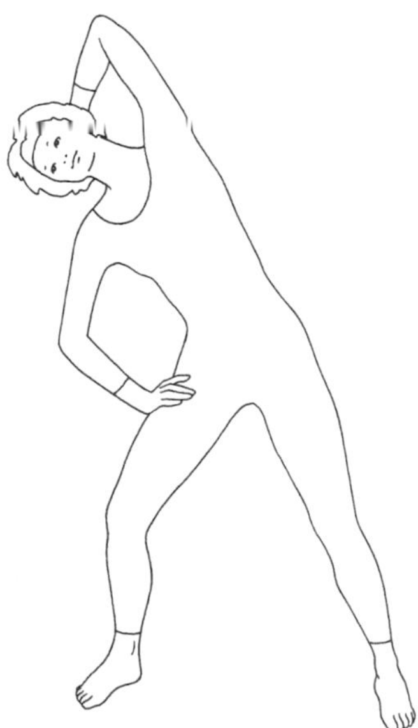

50 SEATED OVERHEAD STRETCH

Sit up straight, balancing on your sit bones. Touch the soles of your feet together with your feet six to eight inches in front of your hips. Place your left fingertips on the floor beside you and your right hand behind your head. Lift your right elbow to the ceiling as you incline your torso to the left. Make sure to keep your right hip on the floor. Switch sides.

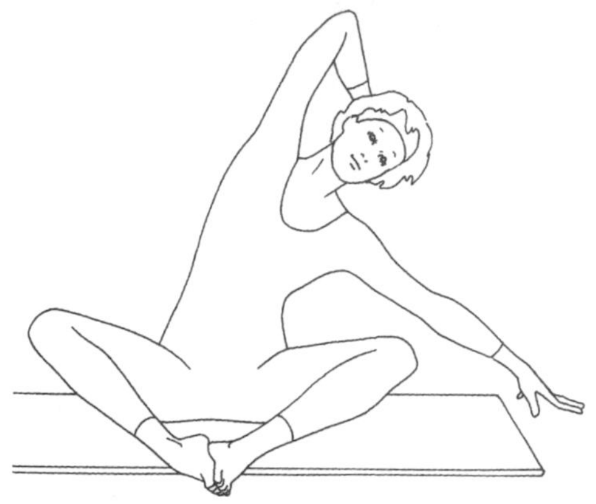

51 STRADDLE OVERHEAD STRETCH

Sitting on the floor, open your legs in a V shape. If you can't do this while keeping your back upright, either bring your legs closer together or do exercise #50 instead. To stretch to the left, first rotate your torso so your chest faces your right leg, *then* bend your torso over your left leg. Place your left hand or elbow on the floor or below your left knee. Extend your right arm overhead and to the left, keeping your right shoulder down. Slowly lift your torso back to vertical. Switch sides.

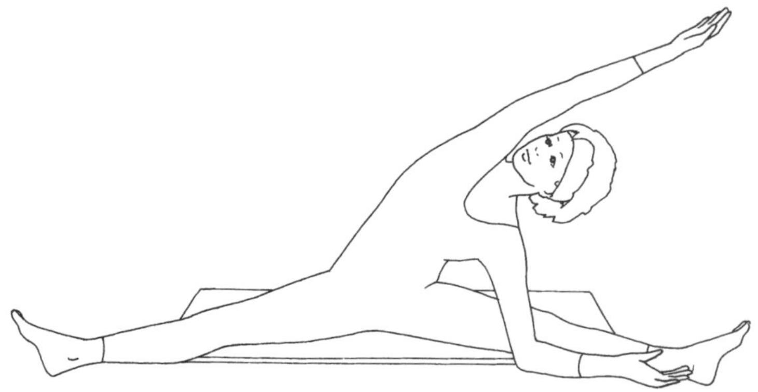

UPPER BACK

If you slump forward, you stretch your upper-back muscles—but not in a healthy way or through a full range of motion. Consciously stretching these muscles, however, will increase your spine's range of motion. Flexibility in your spine gives the vertebrae greater "shock absorption," making them better able to withstand running, jumping, and other jarring motions. The stretches in this section involve your "lats," rhomboids, trapezius muscles, and shoulders. Some include the lower back.

52 HUG YOURSELF

You can do this standing or seated. Grab hold of your back *under* your shoulder blades. Give yourself a strong bear hug and pull your shoulder blades *away* from each other with your hands. Drop your head forward to relieve neck tension at the same time. Keep your shoulders down. For best results, synchronize this movement with your breath this way: inhale, hug, exhale, drop shoulders, drop neck, and hold.

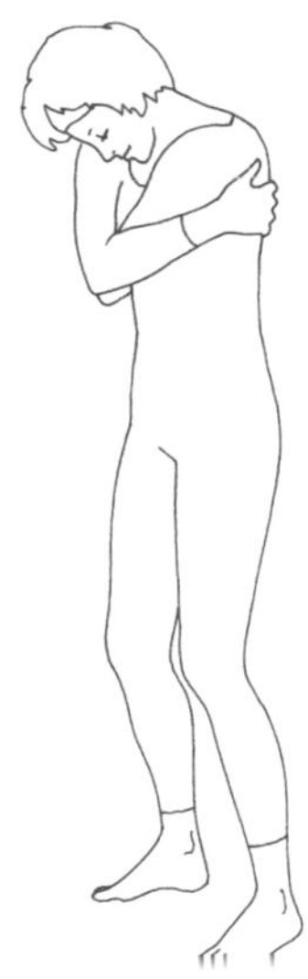

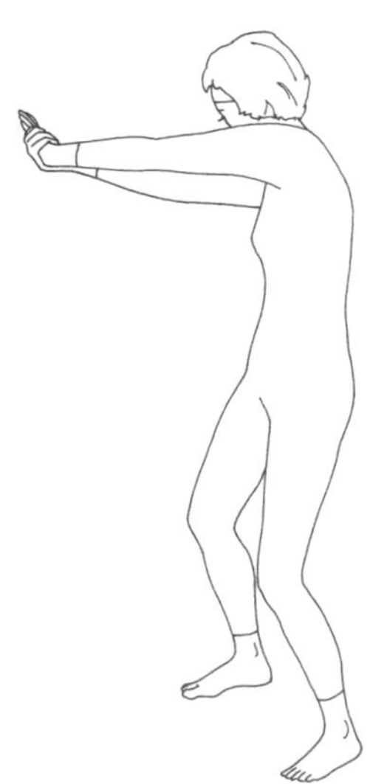

53 SIDE WRIST PULL

This works best standing. Cross your left arm over the midline of your body and hold the left wrist in your right hand down at the level of your hips. Start the stretch with a bent left arm. Slowly straighten, pull, and lift it up to shoulder height, as pictured. Feel this stretch originate in your back, *not* your shoulders, and don't pull too hard on the shoulder joint. Switch sides.

54 ALL-FOURS TWIST

On your hands and knees, move your right arm under your left and rest your right shoulder on the floor. Your weight should be resting on your right shoulder and the right side of your head. For a deeper stretch (in the chest and shoulders), place your left hand on the small of your back. To come out of this, put your left hand on the floor, then the right, and push yourself up. Switch sides.

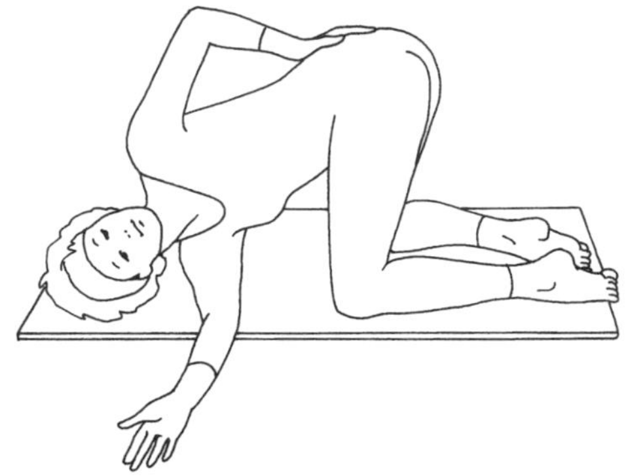

55 SIT-BACK STRETCH

Find some sort of fixed pole, fence, or object that won't topple over if you pull on it. Stand about an arm's length in front of it and take a hip-distance stance with your feet. Hold the pole with both hands and sit your hips back *away* from it (your back should incline forward, as in a squat position). Your weight should rest in your heels and hips. Let your shoulders and upper back stretch and elongate your spine. Keep your head in line with your spine.

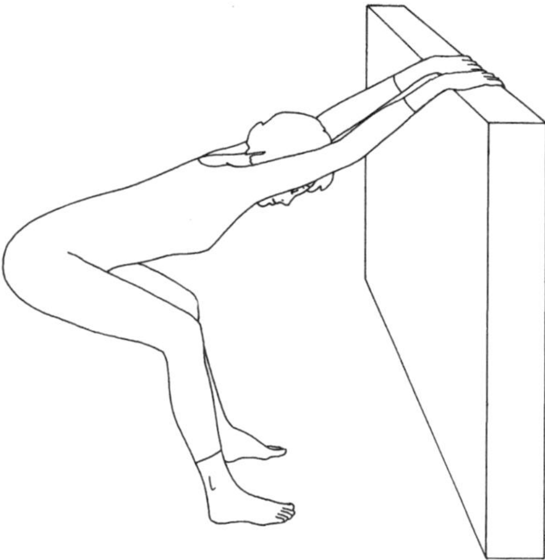

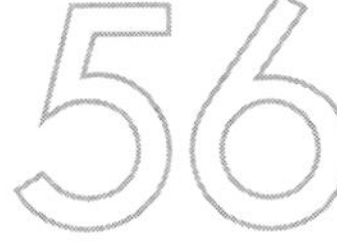

56 ONE-ARM SIT-BACK STRETCH

To get a deeper lat and rhomboid stretch on one side, hold the pole with one hand. Sit your hips back away from it and stretch from tailbone to shoulder, as in stretch #55. To deepen this even further, move your tailbone to the left if holding the pole with your right hand, and vice versa. Again, keep your head in line with your spine. Switch sides.

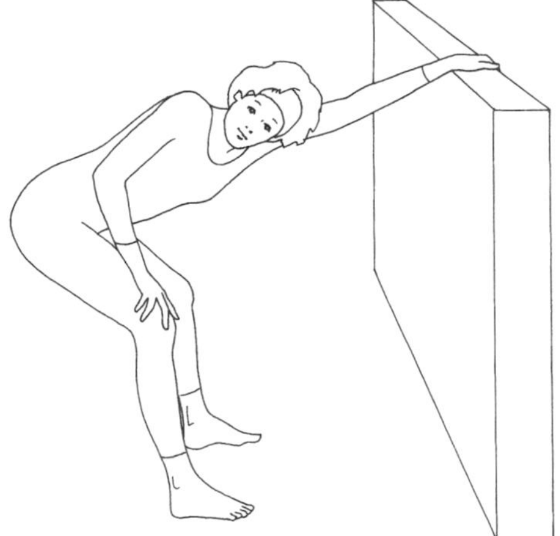

CHEST AND FRONT OF SHOULDERS

Short and tight chest and front shoulder muscles make the chest cave in and the shoulders roll forward. The result is a defeated-looking posture. The funny thing is, you can get this way by being either too strong or too weak. Weight lifters and swimmers who work their pecs but don't stretch them put their shoulders in a state of perpetual internal rotation and cause this posture. People who do no upper-body strengthening work frequently end up with short pectorals as well. Because they also have weak upper-back and rear-shoulder muscles, these muscles aren't strong enough to pull their posture upright.

Stretching can help in both cases. The best chest and shoulder stretches both lift the arm and externally rotate the shoulder (your shoulders pull back to let the chest open and the palms of your hands turn up). It's also important to keep the shoulders down and pulled back while you stretch your chest—otherwise, you will fail to get a good stretch. Holding your arms at different heights will also stretch different parts of your chest and shoulders.

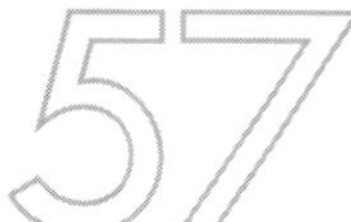

HANDS BEHIND YOUR HEAD

This is a great one to do when you've been sitting too long working over a computer, and it can be done seated or standing. Lace your fingers together with palms out. Put them behind your head and rest your head in your hands. Tilt your head back slightly, lift your chest up, and look at the ceiling. Let your elbows fall open with a little assistance from gravity.

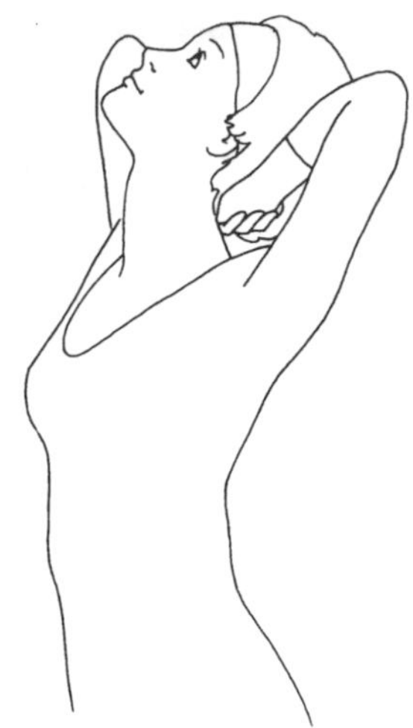

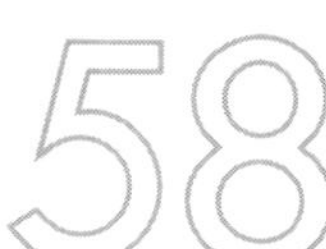

ARMS LOW

Do this one standing. Lace your fingers together and clasp your hands behind your back with palms together. Gently pull your hands down to the floor (to "depress" your shoulder joints). Then, keeping your shoulders down, lift your arms and chest up at the same time. Be conscious of your lower-back and abdominal muscles. Keep your lower back in neutral. There's no need to arch the spine here. This is a great stretch to do in the shower with the warm water running down your back.

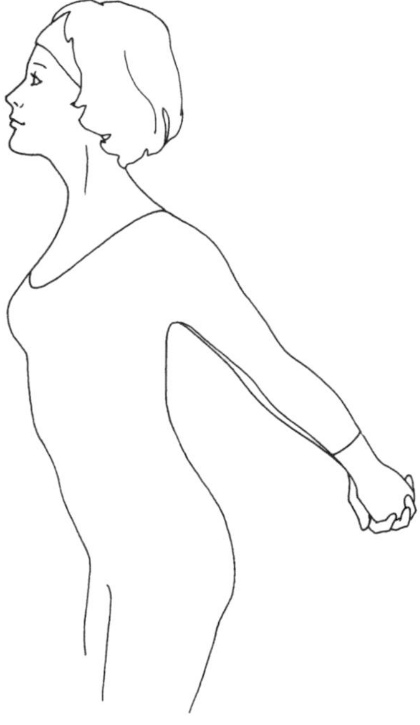

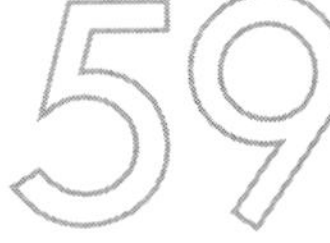

DOORWAY STRETCH

If you've got short arms, you may need to find a narrow doorway. Stand inside a doorway, lift your arms, and bend your elbows at a 90-degree angle. Slowly move forward through the doorway until your elbows end up slightly behind you. Make sure you use your stomach and lower-back muscles to hold you in the proper position.

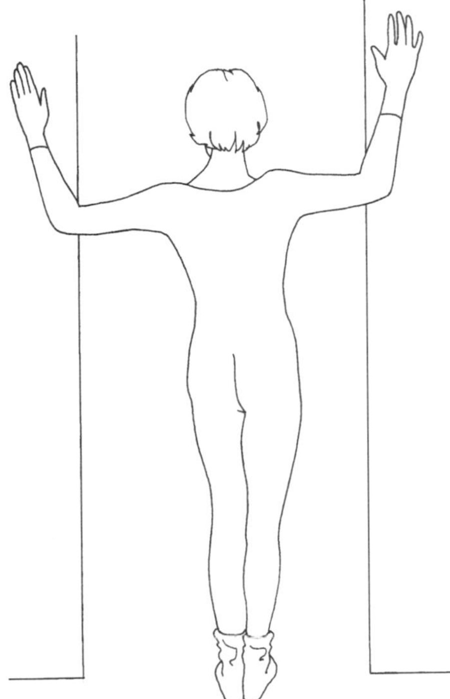

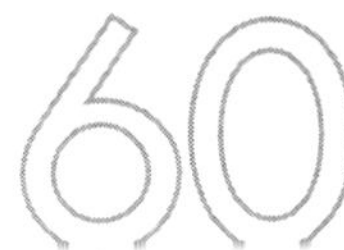

ON-YOUR-KNEES CHAIR STRETCH

Kneel on the floor in front of a chair (make sure the chair won't slip or roll away). Place your elbows on the chair and place your torso parallel to the floor. Slowly lower your head below the chair. It's okay to gently arch your spine here. The force of gravity combined with the weight of your body will give you a good stretch. Also, the higher your chair, the harder this is. Use caution when trying this for the first time.

SHOULDERS AND ARMS

The shoulder joint is one of the most unstable joints in the body. Because the bones inside the shoulder are relatively small, the muscles and ligaments have to provide much of the stability. Also, the shoulders are involved in just about every upper-body motion there is. They lift up and press down (elevate and depress), move forward and back (protract and retract), rotate forward and back, hold steady as you raise your arms (abduct), cross your arms over your body (adduct), and bend and straighten your arms (flex and extend). Since they get high usage but have a relatively weak design, it's no wonder they're so vulnerable to injury.

Lots of people have shoulder problems. Swimmers, weight lifters, tennis players, and gymnasts in particular suffer from "impingement syndrome." This painful inflammation inside the joint can be caused by general overuse—but even building larger muscles can limit the range of motion. Another common cause of pain occurs when the shoulder joint pinches the bursa (a little cushioning sac of fluid that pads the joint). Sharp, sudden motions, bad weight-training techniques, and overworking the muscles without rest all contribute to shoulder pain and make it worse.

Stretching the shoulders gives them better resiliency and can increase the pain-free range of motion inside the joint. It's especially important to stretch the shoulders before and after all sports that involve throwing or lifting.

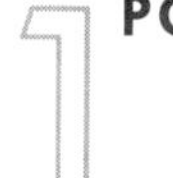

POSTERIOR SHOULDER STRETCH

Standing or sitting, draw one arm across the body and pull it into the body at the elbow. Keep the shoulder down as you do this. Switch sides.

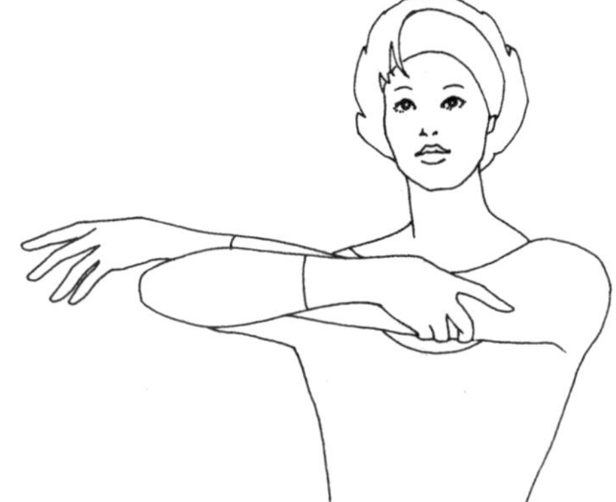

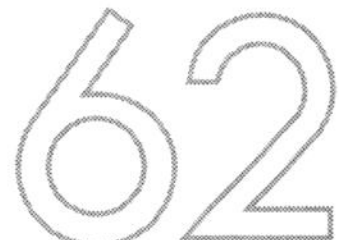

EXTERNAL ROTATOR STRETCH

With one arm above your head and one below, grab hold of a towel, belt, or pole behind your back—or if you're very flexible touch your fingers behind your back. (If you can't touch your fingers, you'll know that your rotators are tight. If the shoulder joint of your higher arm feels tighter, your external rotators are tight on that side. If the shoulder joint of your lower arm feels tighter, your internal rotators are tight on that arm.) Slowly pull down with your lower arm to stretch the external rotators of the top arm. You can proceed to the internal rotator stretch (below) before switching sides.

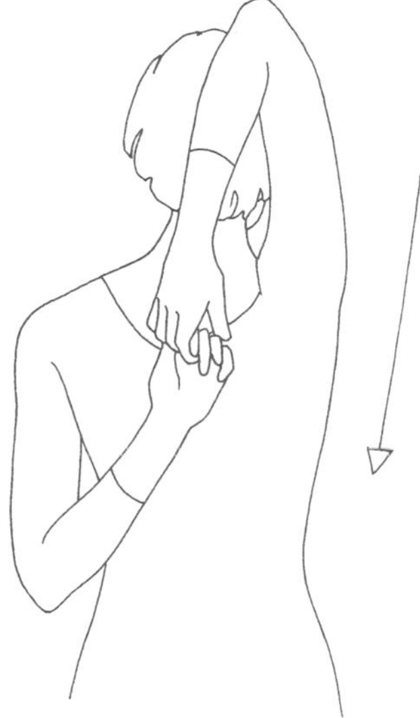

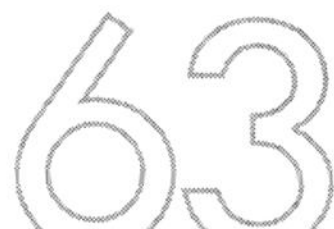

INTERNAL ROTATOR STRETCH

In the same position as above, pull up with the higher arm to stretch the internal rotators of the lower arm. Don't worry if your range of motion is small. Switch sides.

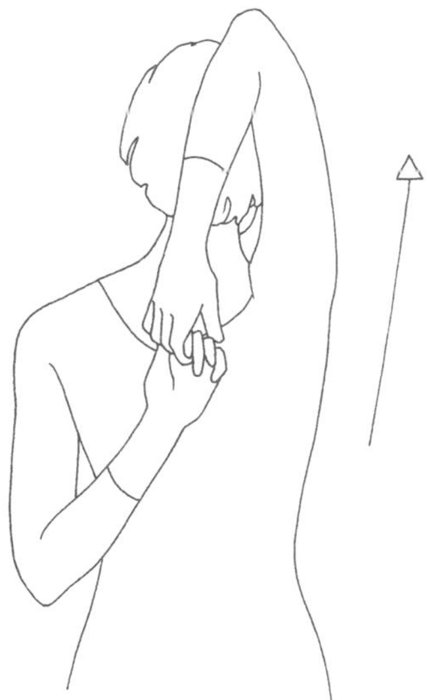

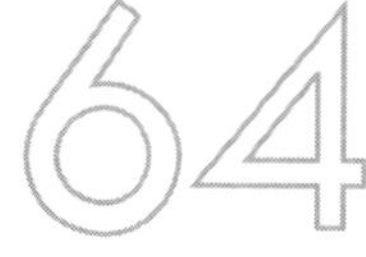

TRICEPS STRETCH

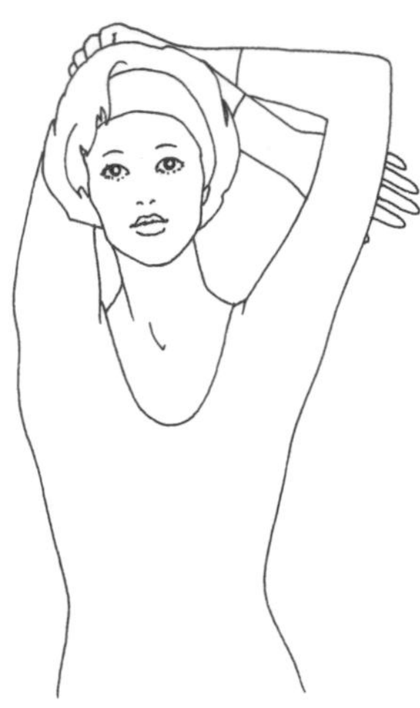

Raise your right arm over your head and hold on to your right elbow with your left hand. Gently pull your right elbow down toward your left shoulder. Remember to keep your right shoulder down. Switch sides.

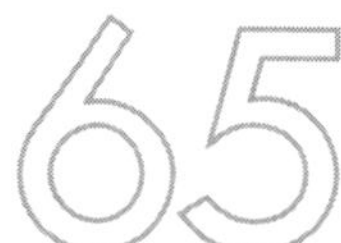

BICEPS STRETCH

Stand facing away from a doorway. Grab hold of the doorjamb with one hand and straighten your arm (incline your torso slightly forward). Your thumb should be pointing down. Slowly and carefully rotate your biceps up toward the ceiling while holding the doorjamb to stretch the biceps. Switch sides.

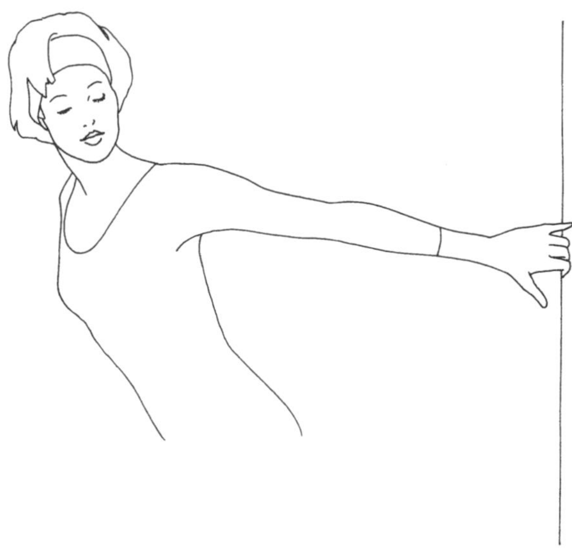

NECK

Exercise caution when stretching your neck. As we mentioned in "Stretching 101," rolling your head in a full circle to stretch your neck is a bad idea. When the head is tilted back and to the side, the weight of the head shifts off the vertebrae and into the small facet joints—which have little weight-bearing capacity. Being in that awkward position can make any common misalignment of the neck vertebrae even worse and compress the nerves that run through the spine.

As also mentioned in "Stretching 101," the extreme neck flexion that you get when doing the yoga plow or shoulder stand is especially dangerous because it puts your full body weight on this delicate part of the spine and can damage ligaments and discs. A non-weight-bearing forward stretch of the head is fine, though. (See stretch #66.) But since age, gravity, and bad posture tend to give people a chronically forward head posture anyway, the back-of-the-neck stretch shouldn't be the *only* neck stretch in your repertoire.

Before you do any neck stretch, pull your chin back to get into neutral posture and be sure to get in and out of each stretch *slowly,* using muscular control.

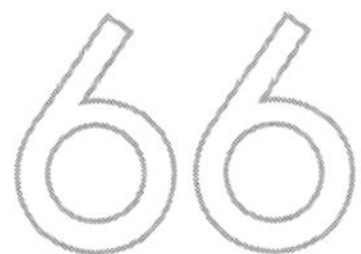

BACK-OF-THE-NECK STRETCH

Lie down with your knees bent and your feet on the floor. Lace your fingers together behind your head and lift your head off the floor so the top of your head curls toward your feet. Keep your shoulders on the floor or you will lose the value of this stretch. You'll feel this in your upper back as well as your neck.

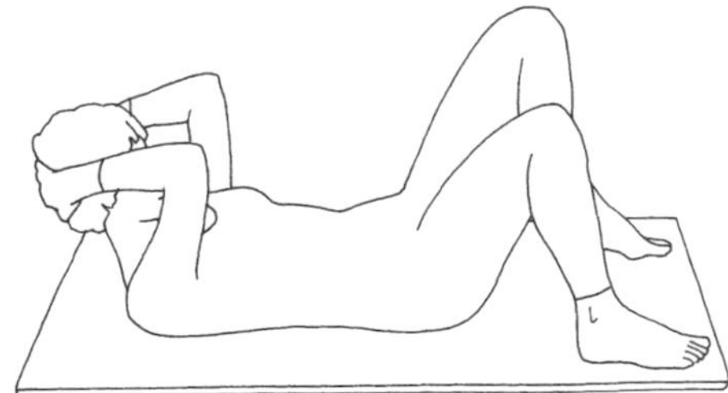

67

LATERAL NECK STRETCH

Place your right hand over your head and on your left ear. Anchor your left shoulder down either by sitting and holding on to the side of a chair or standing and holding a weight in your left hand. Gently pull the right ear to your right shoulder. Switch sides.

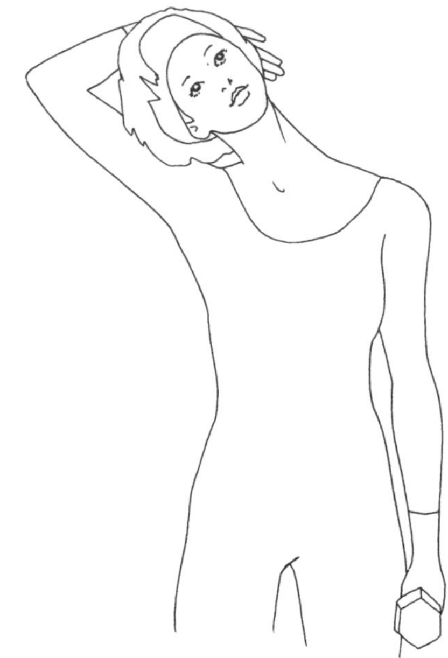

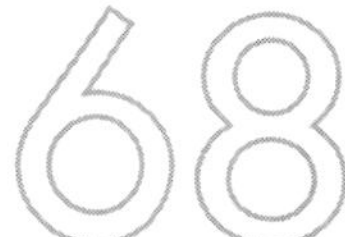

OBLIQUE EXTENSOR STRETCH

Turn your head 45 degrees to the right (halfway between the midline of your body and your right shoulder). Now drop your head down on that same diagonal line. With your right hand, gently pull your head down on the diagonal (if your hair is long enough, it's actually easier to do this by pulling on the hair that grows from the crown of your head). Keep your left shoulder anchored down as in stretch #67, by holding on to either a chair or a dumbbell. Switch sides.

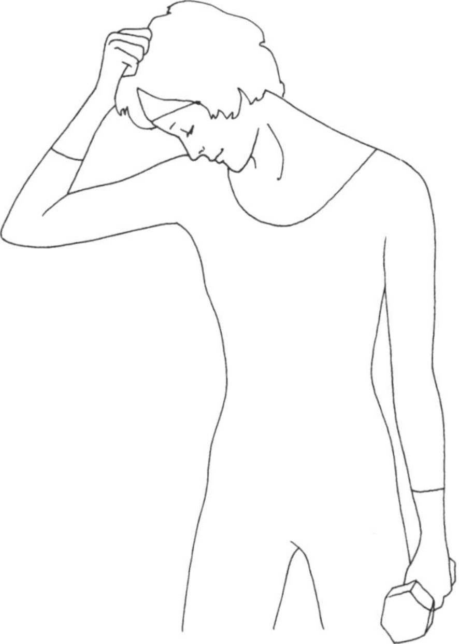

WRISTS AND FINGERS

Repetitive tasks such as working at a computer keyboard all day and playing certain sports can cause carpal tunnel syndrome. Carpal tunnel syndrome is an inflammation of the nerves that run through a "tunnel" in the wrist. When this tunnel becomes inflamed and constricted, the result is pain and numbness in the wrists. Flexibility plays a critical role in both preventing and treating this condition. Flexing the wrists is especially helpful. (See stretch #69.)

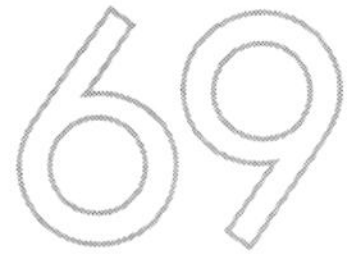

WRIST FLEXOR STRETCH

Hold your left fingers with your right hand and point the left fingers up (palm is out). Gently pull the fingers back toward your body. Switch sides or proceed to the next stretch.

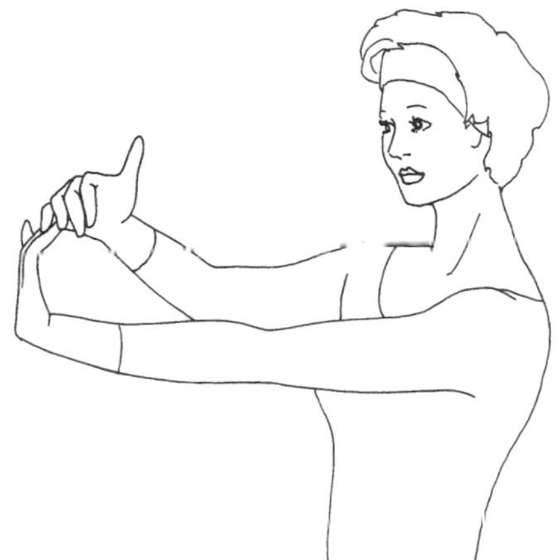

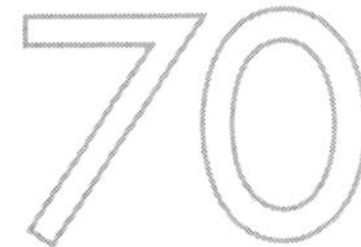

WRIST EXTENSOR STRETCH

Turn the palm toward your body, point the fingers down, and gently pull the fingers back toward your body. Switch sides or do stretches #69 and #70 in succession for your other wrist.

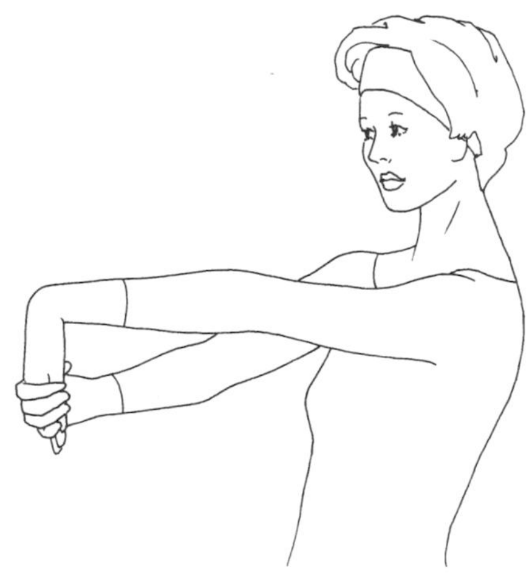

71 WRIST ROTATOR STRETCH

Face your left palm into your chest. Hold it with your right hand and gently rotate the left palm to the left shoulder. The little finger twists out to the left side. Switch sides.

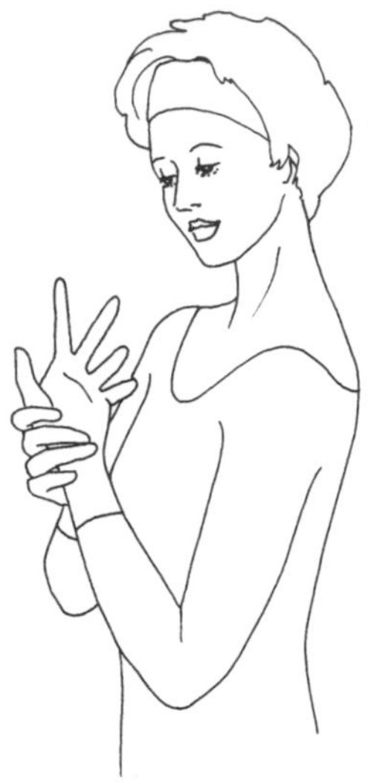

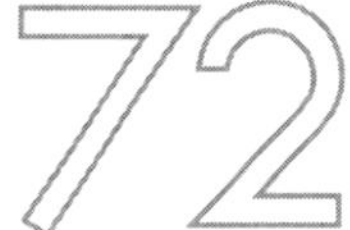

72 FINGER STRETCHES

Turn the left palm to the ceiling and hold your four fingers in your right hand. Gently pull the fingers down toward the floor. Do the same with the thumb. Switch sides.

ANKLES AND FEET

Most of us forget to stretch our ankles and feet—we take them for granted. But have you ever tried to run on cold ankles and feet? It's hard to move! When these muscles are supple, they can absorb the shock of walking and running much better than when they're tight.

You'll need a belt, strap, towel, or rope for most of these stretches. You'll get more flexibility with your shoes off.

73 FLEX AND POINT

Lie on your back, with one knee bent and that foot on the floor. Lift the other leg and loop your strap around your arch. To create better articulation of the little muscles in your feet (especially good for dancers and gymnasts), flex your feet in sequence: pull back the toes, the ball of the foot, and then the heel—and hold. To point your foot, first press the heel, then the ball of the foot, and finally the toe—and hold. With your toes flexed, you'll also stretch your calves. Switch sides.

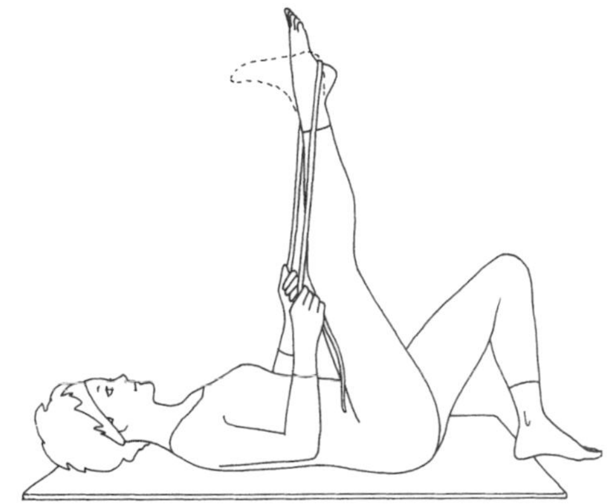

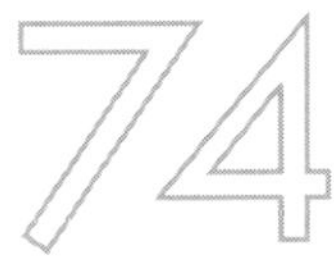

74 TOE GRAB AND SPREAD

You don't need a strap for this one. In the same position as above, with your left leg bent, rotate your right ankle so your right toes face the left and curl your toes under as if you were grabbing a pencil with them. Then rotate your ankle so the toes turn out to the right—and spread your toes. (You might say to yourself while doing this, "In and grab, out and spread.") You can follow this with foot circles in both directions. Switch sides.

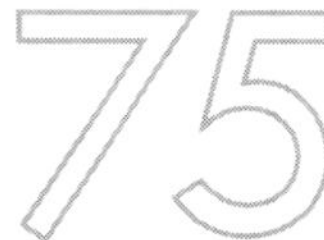

INNER-ANKLE STRETCH

Place the strap around your arch (as in stretch #73), turn the sole of the foot out to your outer thighs, and hold. Proceed to stretch #76.

OUTER-ANKLE STRETCH

With the strap around your arch, turn the sole of the foot in toward your inner thighs to stretch the outside of the ankle (the side that tends to get sprained). Hold. Repeat stretches #75 and #76 with the other foot.

FACE

Stretching your facial muscles can change your whole appearance (at least temporarily) and instantly make you look happier, younger, and more relaxed. Facial muscles are more challenging to stretch than other muscles, since you need to use your hands to create a place to stretch from. Be conscious not to overstretch your skin when you do these. The best time to do them is just after you've applied moisturizer.

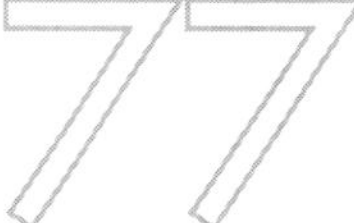

THE JAW

The jaw is the tightest muscle in the body. It was designed to allow you to talk and eat all day without suffering from burning jaws! To stretch your jaw, open your mouth and place your fingertips on your chin. Tilt your head up slightly and gently pull the chin down. You can finish this stretch with a light massage on your jaw muscles. (Some deep-tissue body workers massage the jaw on the *inside* of the mouth—which is quite intense. We recommend you do this by touching the face on the outside.)

BROW STRETCH

Place the palms of your hands in the center of your brow. Gently sweep your hands outward to flatten out the brow. Hold. You can finish this stretch by rubbing your temples with the heel of your hands or your fingertips.

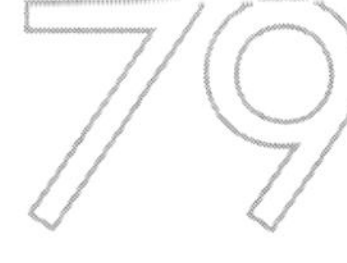

LEMON FACE

Imagine scrunching your face into a tight little ball (as if you just sucked on a lemon). Tensing the muscles this way will prepare them for the next stretch.

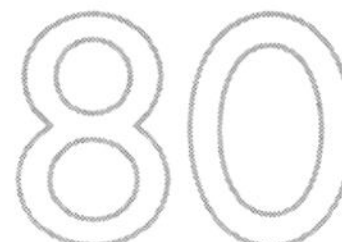

LION FACE

Think of stretching your entire face as much as possible while doing this. Open your eyes and mouth as wide as you can and stick out your tongue. This classic yoga posture stretches your jaw, cheeks, and eyes. It's hard *not* to smile after you do this!

SPECIALTY STRETCHES

POLE

A simple unattached pole adds "structure" to your stretches in a number of ways. It helps hold you in proper alignment, provides a good visual aid if you happen to use it in front of a mirror (it helps you create "clean lines"), and lends a sense of security because it gives you something to hold on to.

The exercise we *don't* recommend with the pole is probably the most common: standing up with the pole behind your shoulders, looped through your arms, and quickly twisting the torso. This is a risky move for the muscles and ligaments around the spine and the ligaments in the knees, especially if you hold your legs straight. If you hold the pole at shoulder height and quickly twist, you build momentum—but the soft tissues in the knees and spine lack the ability to absorb the shock of that motion. To make this move safer, simply hold a stationary twist (see stretch #4) and add a pole. Sitting down while you do this also reduces any risk to the ligaments in the knees.

You can use a broomstick, closet dowel, cane, or umbrella as your pole.

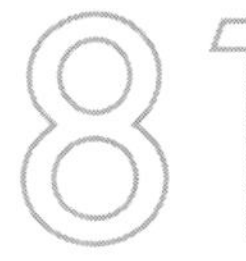

81 CHEST AND FRONT-OF-SHOULDER STRETCH

This also stretches your shoulder's external rotators. Stand with your legs together. Take a slightly wider than shoulder-width grip on the pole and hold it in front of you with your palms facing down. Carefully lift the pole up and behind your head. Remain aware of your lower-body alignment. Keep your stomach muscles tucked in and your lower-back muscles contracted to avoid arching your lower back.

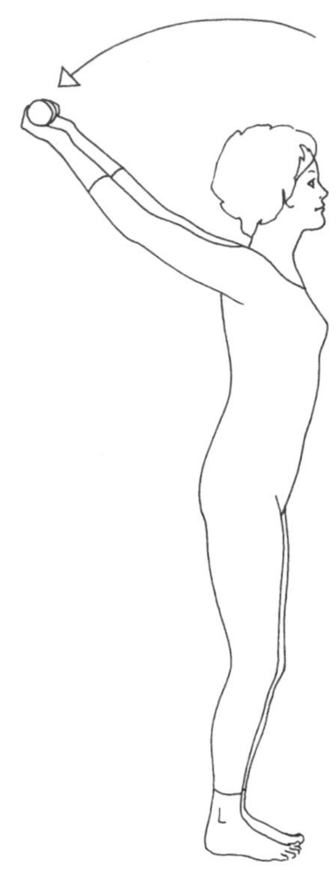

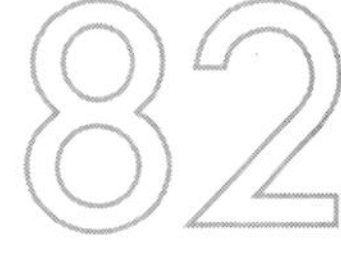

82 ROUND-THE-WORLD SHOULDER STRETCH

Stand with your legs together. Hold the pole behind your hips with a wider-than-shoulder-width grip. Your palms should be down and your thumbs facing out. Slowly lift your arms up behind your head (you'll feel your shoulders rotate in the shoulder joint). You'll probably hit a "sticking point" where it's hard to lift it further. (Don't force it!)

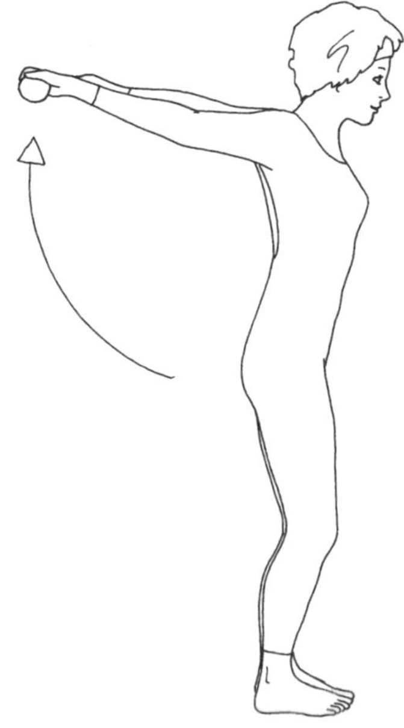

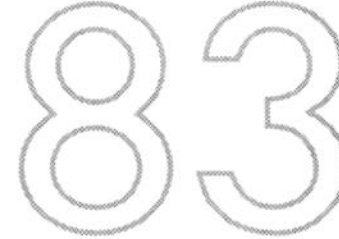

83 SIDE TORSO STRETCH

Place the pole on your shoulders and hold it with both hands. Begin the stretch by tilting to your left side. Draw your left elbow into your side to help stabilize your torso, and straighten your right arm overhead so that the pole is at least vertical or creates a deeper, diagonal line. Switch sides.

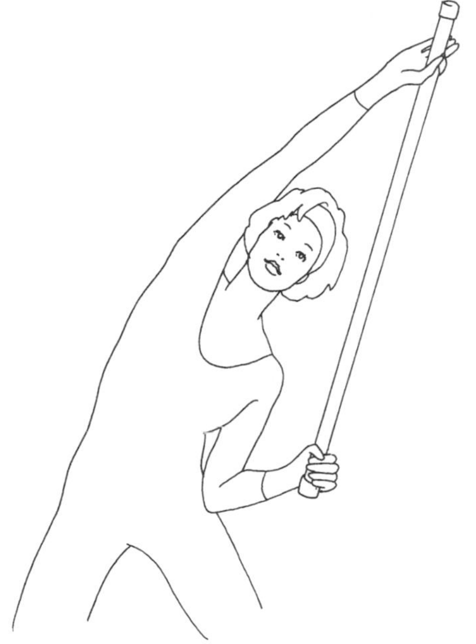

84 HUG A POLE

With the pole held horizontal in front of you, cross your arms over your chest and hold on to the pole so that your hands are as far apart as possible. Pull both hands in toward the middle as you maintain your grip on the pole. The exercise stretches the trapezius, the rhomboids (upper-back muscles), and the rear part of the shoulders.

BALLET BARRE

A ballet barre is a versatile and effective stretching tool. If you don't have access to one, try a moderately low wall or even playground equipment. Here are three easy, classic inner-thigh and torso stretches.

85 INNER-THIGH STRETCH

You can do these next three stretches all on one side before switching legs (skip any you can't do, of course). If you are not very, very flexible, start with a low stool or bench before progressing to a barre. Stand facing the barre with your heels touching and turn your toes out (at two o'clock and ten o'clock). Lift your right leg and rest your ankle on the barre or wall. Keep your torso vertical. Bend your left knee slightly to stretch the inner thigh. If your inner thighs aren't warm, you can do a few pliés: bend and straighten your supporting knee a few times. Make sure your supporting knee doesn't shoot out over your toe. If it does, scoot your left foot further to the left. To deepen the stretch, slide your right leg along the barre to the right.

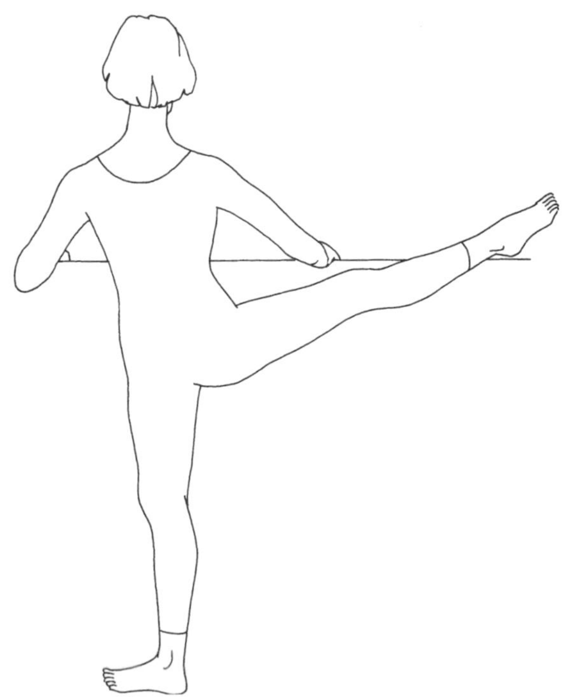

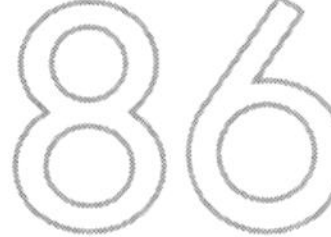

INNER-THIGH AND TORSO STRETCH

If you slid your leg along the barre, bring it back to the starting position. With a vertical torso and your right leg lifted, place your right hand on the barre and lift your left arm overhead to the right.

INNER-THIGH AND OPPOSITE TORSO STRETCH

Return your torso to a vertical position and, this time, place your left hand on the barre and lift your right arm overhead to the left. Change legs, return to stretch #85, and repeat the series.

HANGING AND INVERSION

You can create some very clever stretches in the gym, at the playground, or anyplace you find bars and benches. Be advised: these stretches are for "normal," healthy adults. Do not do them if you have any of the following conditions:

- If you have a shoulder injury, avoid hanging all your weight off your arms (especially one arm), as in stretches #88 and #89.
- If you have glaucoma or hypertension, are on blood thinners such as aspirin, or have a serious back problem, avoid all inverted stretches (whether you're on an angle or completely vertical). Hanging upside down can increase blood pressure, pulse rate, and the pressure inside your eyeballs. (There have been reported cases of blood vessels in the eye rupturing when someone with these conditions hung upside down.)
- If you are pregnant, avoid hanging and inversion, since falling is a big risk.

But if you have none of these concerns, hanging upside down doesn't present any problems. When you're upside down, the blood "rushes to your head," but your brain has a self-protective mechanism that actually prevents it from getting filled with too much blood. Still, hanging with your head below your heart takes some getting used to. Don't stay down for long at first, and get up slowly to avoid feeling dizzy or blacking out! There *are* some benefits to inversion or we wouldn't present it here. Hanging upside down *can*, to some extent, alleviate and prevent back pain. Changing your relationship with gravity elongates the spine, reduces pressure on the nerves that pass through the spine, and increases blood flow and therefore can relieve nervous and muscular tension.

Several types of fancy inversion equipment have slowly been creeping out of the physical therapists' offices and into homes. There are whole catalogs and stores devoted to back swings, hanging chairs, gravity boots, and other devices. Although these can offer relief in very imaginative ways, you can also stick with simple gym and playground equipment to get your inversion fix. Ideally, however, you should add hanging and inversion stretches under the guidance of a qualified physical therapist.

But if you're relatively fit and eager to give it a try, go ahead, and proceed with caution. Try some of the easier angles (a slight decline bench, for instance). Don't use gravity boots. (They are illegal in some states and can cause knee, ankle, and back discomfort. We don't recommend them or show them here.) As with all things, ease your way both in and out of these positions.

A final word on inversion. In some yoga traditions, women are advised against hanging their heads below their hips while menstruating because that puts the body against the natural down and outward blood flow of this time. Some women find inverted postures uncomfortable while they are menstruating. However, going into a slightly inverted posture (such as stretch #7) for 10 seconds should cause no discomfort.

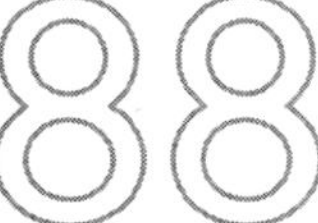

88 THE TWO-HANDED HANG

To stretch your upper back and lats, grab on to a suspended horizontal bar with palms out, hands approximately shoulder-width apart. You can do this with your feet on a bench or keep your legs on the floor if you can reach. In either position, let your tailbone hang to the floor. Contract your abdominal muscles so that your lower back rounds slightly. For a deeper stretch, let all your weight hang off your arms and pull your knees to your chest.

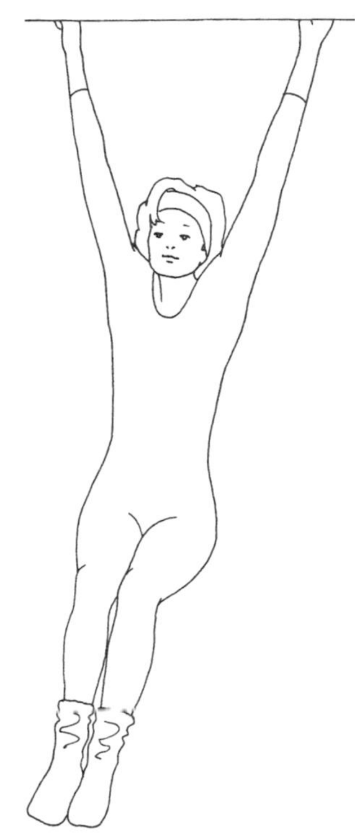

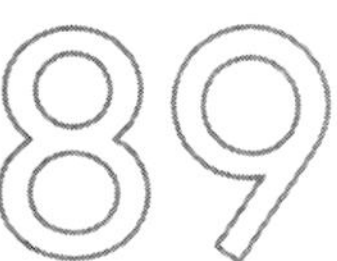

89 THE ONE-HANDED HANG

This offers a more intense stretch than #88, since you're hanging your entire weight off one arm and therefore stretching one side of the torso. Again, put your feet on the floor. (Don't lift your feet. That's a bit much for most people's shoulders.) You can shift weight into either side of your pelvis to stretch your lower-back and hip muscles. You can also rotate your torso forward a bit to stretch your internal shoulder rotators, then slightly back to stretch your external rotators. Switch sides.

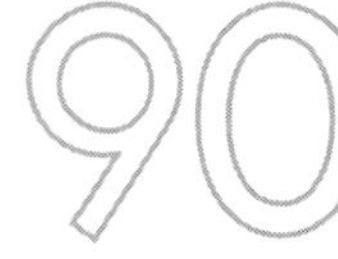

THE HYPEREXTENSION-BENCH STRETCH

In most gyms you can find a "hyperextension bench" where you work your lower-back muscles. This is also a good place to stretch these muscles. Older benches will put your torso into a vertical posture, while newer ones will incline your torso more on a diagonal. (The newer ones are easier on the spine for beginners, but many master stretchers and lifters prefer the old-fashioned bench.) Secure your feet under the pads, making sure your hipbones hang beyond the hip pad, and slowly lower your head to the floor. Let your arms hang forward and straight. If this bothers your knees at all, bend them slightly (i.e., don't lock your knees).

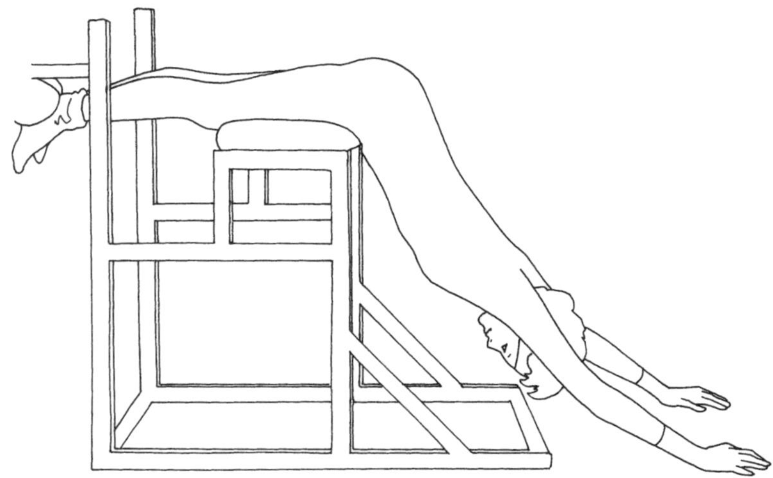

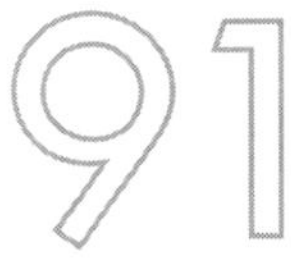

THE DECLINE-BENCH TOTAL-SURRENDER STRETCH

Carefully position yourself on your back on a slanted bench and slowly lower your head below your hips (take about 20 seconds to do this). Decline benches usually have a place to secure your feet and a handy knob you can grab to help pull yourself up. Some declines also have a pad under your knees (easier on the knees than straight

benches). Let your arms stretch down to the floor. It feels good to let your lower-back arch and to lift your chest to the ceiling. You can safely curl up to your seated position *if* you take about 20 seconds to do so and roll up one vertebra at a time.

BALL STRETCHES

The big ball gets our vote as the best all-around stretching tool. Stretching over a ball not only feels great but also contributes more than a stretch. Every time you balance on the ball, you work the stabilizing muscles in your back, abdominals, shoulders, and hips. These stabilizing muscles help you stand up straight and move through the world with greater ease and grace.

The big ball began its life as a rehab tool but has since moved into the general fitness arena. If you're thinking of investing in a ball, try out a few different sizes (they also come in an elliptical shape) to see which suits you best. Space prohibits us from showing the many nonstretching exercises you can do with a ball, but several books and tapes on the market show these and more. Our favorite source for purchasing educational materials and stretch balls in all sizes is Fitness Wholesale, 1-888-396-7337, or *http://www.fitnesswholesale.com* on the Web.

Don't be afraid to experiment with finding the most comfortable and effective positions for your body. *Slowly* roll the ball into position (don't let it roll out from under you!), and try holding a posture, then moving it an inch or two in any direction to feel how that changes the stretch. Once you've hit on a good spot, stay there for at least 10 seconds to get the most out of it. These stretches are listed in order so you can move easily from one position to the next.

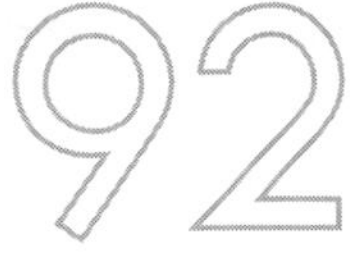

HUG A BALL

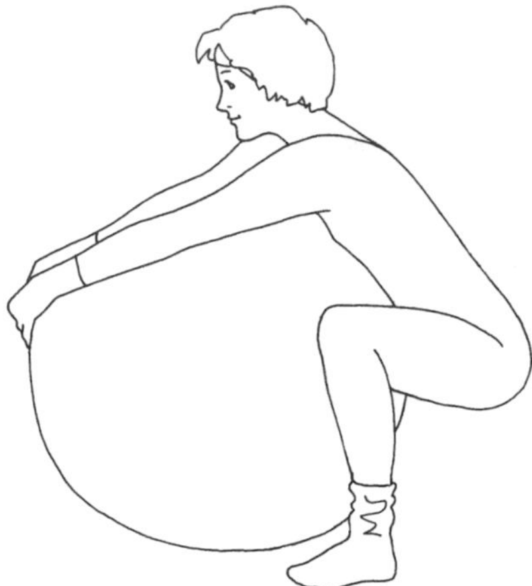

Straddle the ball between both legs and lower your hips down toward the floor (but don't sit). Hug your arms around the ball to support your body. Adjust your legs so that your feet are flat on the floor and your knees line up over your ankles. Keep a good grip on the ball so it doesn't roll away from you and send you back onto your buttocks. This stretches your lower and upper back and also your buttocks and calves.

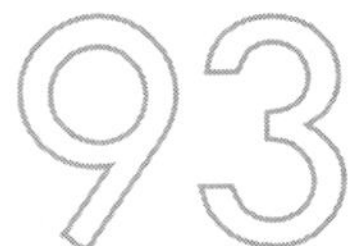

PYRAMID

Roll your torso forward onto the ball so your hips rest on top of the ball—and become the highest point of your body. Rest your hands and feet on the floor. Your arms and legs can be slightly bent or straight, depending on the size of the ball, your flexibility, and the length of your limbs. This stretches your lower back, while gravity assists in stretching your upper back. This also helps develop stabilizing strength in your torso and shoulders.

DOWNWARD-FACING BALANCE

While resting on the ball (as in stretch #93), walk your hands forward along the floor and lift your legs so they are even with your torso or, for a deeper stretch, slightly higher. Both your legs and arms can be straight or bent. Focus on stretching the entire front of the body: the chest, abdominals, and hip flexors. This also adds stability in the abdominals, lower back, hips, and shoulders.

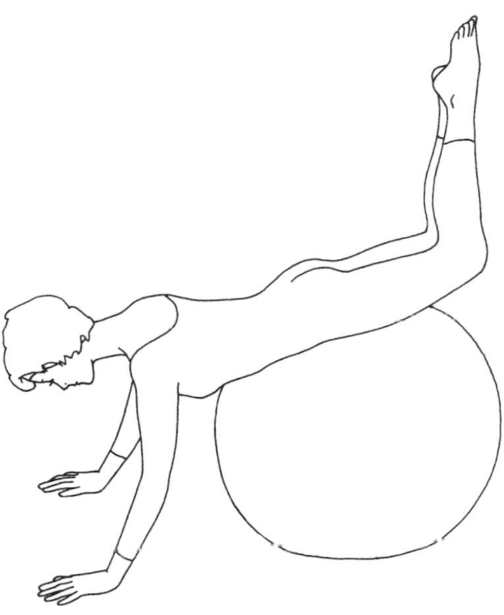

95 INNER-THIGH STRETCH

Open your legs and bend your knees as you roll the ball slightly back to straddle the ball between your legs. Perch on the ball (as if laying an egg!). This stretches the inner thighs and lower back and adds stability in the torso, hips, and shoulders.

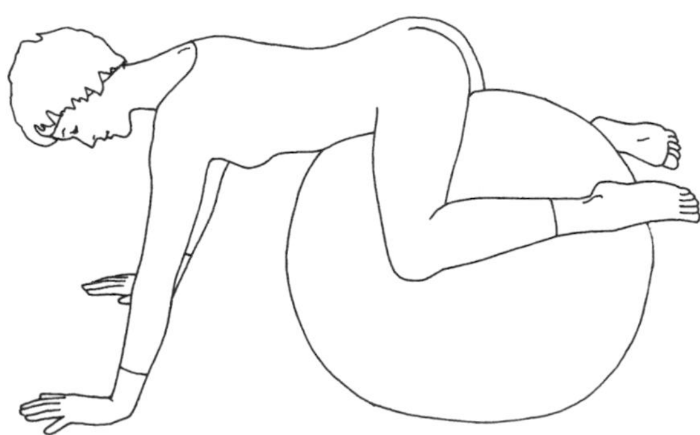

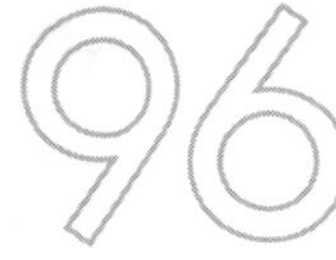

DEEPEST BACK STRETCH

Do this only if you have something directly in front of you to hold on to that's fixed and won't move if you pull on it. (A ballet barre or fixed pole will do. Otherwise, skip it.) Straddle the ball while facing the barre. As you hold the barre, let your arms straighten and sit back into your hips and tailbone while straddling the ball. Go for the maximum lower- and upper-back stretch.

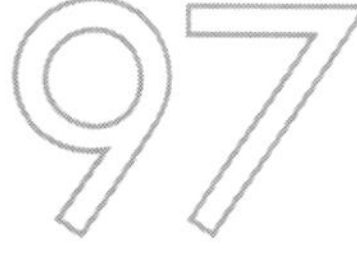

GROIN AND CHEST STRETCH

Get up from your last stretch and sit on the ball with your knees bent, legs wider than your hips and your feet flat on the floor. Slowly start to walk your feet forward, grab hold of the sides of the ball with your hands, and slide your back down the ball. As you get to the deepest part of the stretch (in a squat position), lift one arm from the side of the ball to over the ball and hold it there firmly. Keep your feet flat and far enough in front of you so your knees don't jut out over your toes. This stretches the chest, torso, inner thighs, and buttocks.

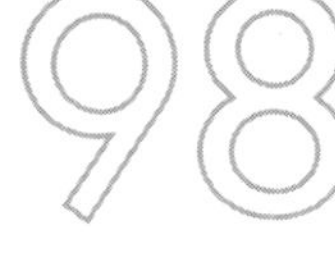

UPWARD BALANCE

Slowly adjusting from stretch #97, press into your feet and roll your torso back onto the ball so that your chest is facing the ceiling. Keep your knees bent at a 90-degree angle to begin the stretch. Once you feel stable perched on the ball, extend your arms overhead. To deepen the stretch, you can straighten your legs. This stretches the chest, front part of the shoulders, abdominals, and hip flexors.

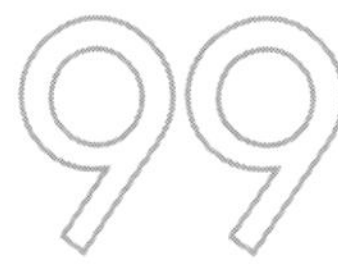

SIDEWAYS BALANCE

This is a little tricky to get into, but it's a great stretch for the whole side of your body. Start seated on the floor, next to the ball. Rise up onto the knee closest to the ball and roll your torso on a diagonal line across the ball. Be sure to hold the ball tight with your supporting arm and find your balance before taking this further. Then slowly extend your top arm and, for a deeper hip stretch, straighten your top leg. For a maximum torso stretch, look up at your extended arm.

WATER STRETCHES

Water is a forgiving place to stretch. In chest-high water, you lose 80 percent of your body weight and you don't feel the same old effects of gravity holding you down. In fact, because the body tends to rise (body fat is actually what makes us buoyant), most of us can float our way to flexibility. Water stretches are good for older, injured, tight people, as well as for the very fit, because water lets you take your stretches further without a struggle.

The ideal water temperature for stretching is at least 82 degrees. It's hard to relax your muscles when you're shivering in cold water (and cold muscles don't stretch as far).

It's best to have something to hold on to while you stretch in the water, in order to stabilize your torso. (You can stretch while floating if you have good stabilizing strength in your torso and abdominals. See stretch #106.) For most of these stretches you can hold the wall or use the pool steps or ladder. You can even hang off the diving board.

To take your stretches further, add additional buoyant cuffs around your ankles or wrists (you can buy kids' "water wings" or other buoyant devices in swimmers' catalogs and in some sporting goods stores). These help buoy your limbs, which makes stretching more effective.

100 HOLD THE LEG

For inner thighs. Stand with one side close to the wall. Lift the outside leg, keeping your supporting knee bent. Your lifted leg shouldn't be directly out to the side but slightly in front of you. Without cuffs on your ankles, hold on under the lifted knee. With cuffs you can let the leg float on its own. To stretch both inner thighs at the same time, bend your supporting knee. Switch sides.

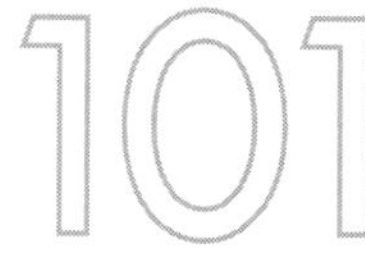

CLIMB THE WALL

For the lower back, hamstrings, and calves. Turn and face the wall. (It's easier to hold on if your pool has a slight ledge. If not, press your palms flat down onto the pool edge to give yourself a counterweight. Or you can hold on to a ladder and place your feet on the rungs.) Bend both knees and put the soles of both feet on the wall, with one leg higher than the other. Let your tailbone drop down and sit your hips back away from the wall. You can do this with or without cuffs. For a deeper hamstring stretch, try to straighten the lower leg. Switch sides.

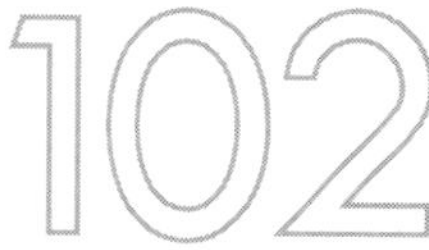

STEP STRETCH

For the hip flexors, quads, and calves. If your pool has stairs, put one foot on the highest stair you can comfortably reach and keep the sole of the foot down. With no stairs, put your foot on the wall and face the wall. Straighten your supporting leg and angle it slightly behind your torso, keeping the heel down (to stretch the calf on the back leg). Slowly bring your hips forward to stretch the hip flexors and quads on the front leg. This is another one you can do easily without cuffs. Switch sides.

103 ANKLE-ACROSS-THE-KNEE STRETCH

With your back against the wall, extend your arms along the pool edge so you can hold yourself up. (Be aware, however, that if the water level in your pool is low, this could stress your shoulders.) Cross your left foot or ankle on your right knee (as below) and pull both knees to your chest. This is easier to do if you're wearing buoyant cuffs. Without the cuffs, make a greater effort to tuck both knees to the chest. This stretches the buttocks and lower back. Do the next stretch before switching sides.

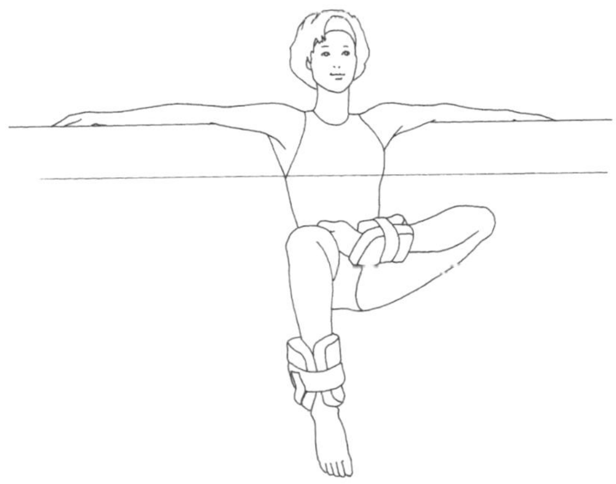

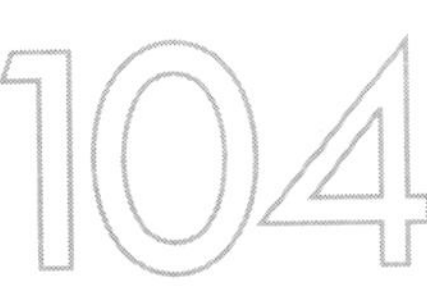

HIP STRETCH

Keep your left ankle crossed over your right knee as above. Straighten your right leg and slide it along the wall to the left so it forms a horizontal line parallel to the pool floor. This will point your left knee upward. Relax your weight down into your right hip. This stretches the outer hip and torso.

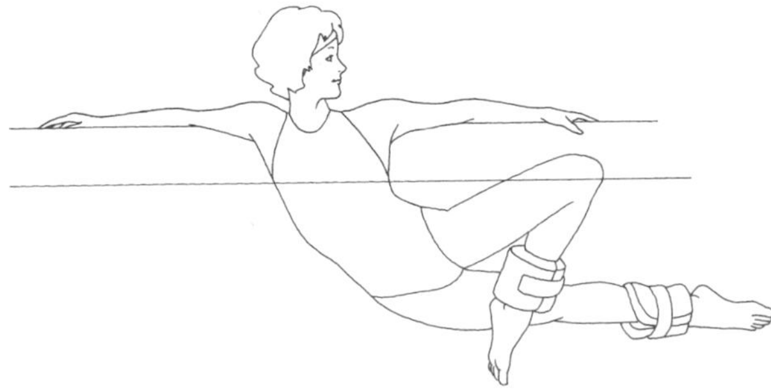

105 DIVING BOARD STRETCH

Hang on to a diving board for this abdominal strengthener and lower-back stretch. Start with your torso straight. Then move both knees through the water to your left shoulder. Once they've gone as far as they can, turn the knees and take them to the right shoulder. To make this harder (and add a strengthening exercise for the abdominals), use straighter legs while you move them in the water to the other side. Buoyant cuffs will make the abdominal strengthening exercise harder but will make it easier to hold your final stretches. After completing as many reps as you want, hold the final position with your knees to your shoulder for an oblique and lower-back stretch. Switch sides.

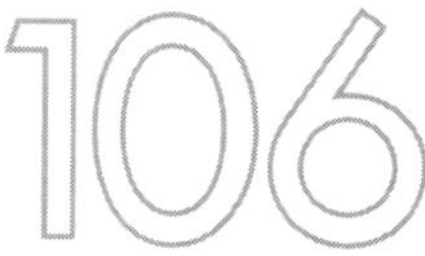

106 FREE-FLOATING INNER-THIGH STRETCH

This one's definitely easier to do with cuffs on. (You could also do it holding a pair of buoyant dumbbells or a kickboard under each elbow, but it won't be as effective for your legs.) Open your legs and lift your feet off the pool bottom. Pull your knees up toward the surface and relax your inner thighs. To maintain this position for any period of time, you'll have to "scull your hands" in the water in front of you (i.e., stir the water) to stay afloat. This will work your torso stabilizers. Don't give up if you don't get it right away.

STRETCHES FOR LIFE

MORNING STRETCHES

Stretching first thing in the morning is natural. (You've probably seen dogs and cats do it!) It not only wakes up body and mind, it "resets" the resting length of your muscles for the rest of the day. In other words, morning stretches make your muscles longer, more relaxed, and better able to take on all kinds of tasks.

Before you stretch, warm up with a short walk or some shoulder rolls, hip rotations, leg swings, and the like. You can skip the warm up and simply stretch—even while still in bed—but you won't be able to stretch as far. However you do it, be gentle, and don't expect to be your most flexible first thing in the morning.

Hug knees to chest (lower back)
STRETCH #1

Ankle on the knee (buttocks, hips, and lower back)
STRETCH #14

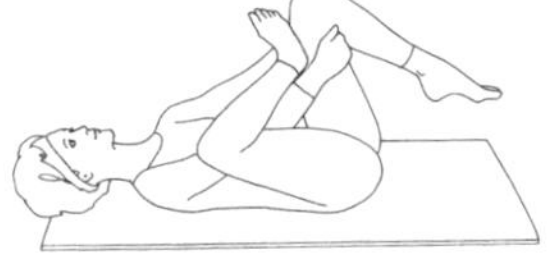

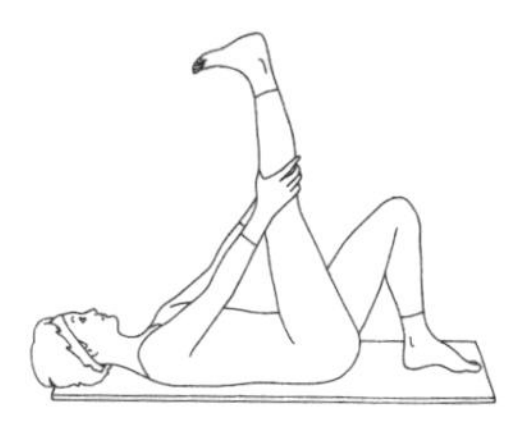

Leg-up hamstring stretch
STRETCH #27

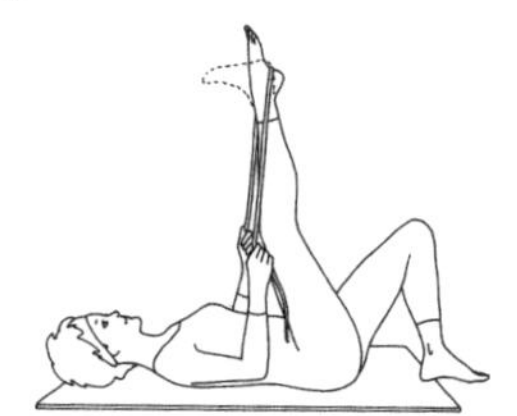

Flex and point (ankles and feet)
STRETCH #73

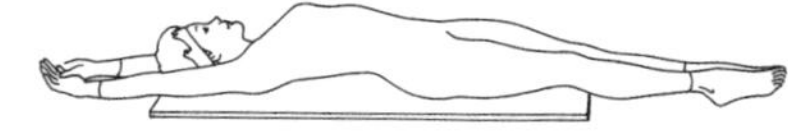

Full-body stretch (abdominals)
STRETCH #45

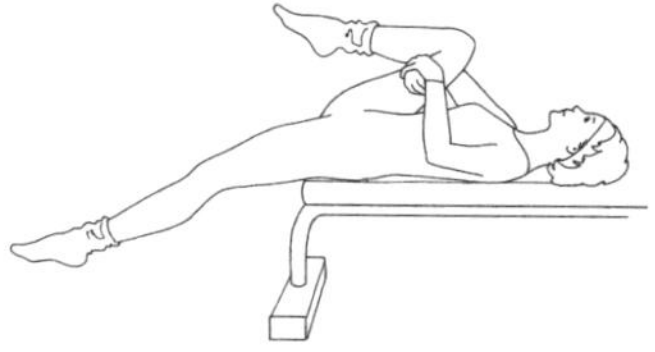

Bench hip flexor stretch
STRETCH #24

On-your-back quad stretch
STRETCH #17

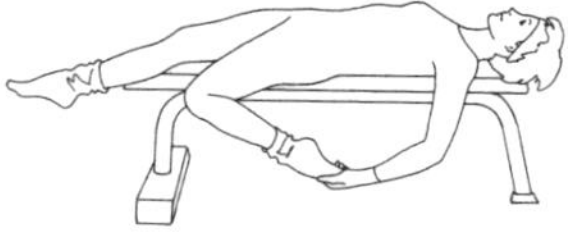

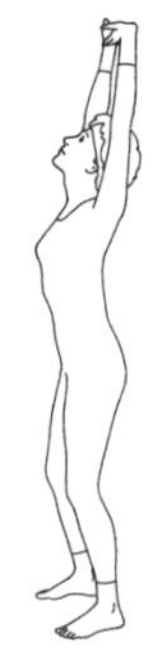

Overhead stretch (obliques and torso)
STRETCH #48

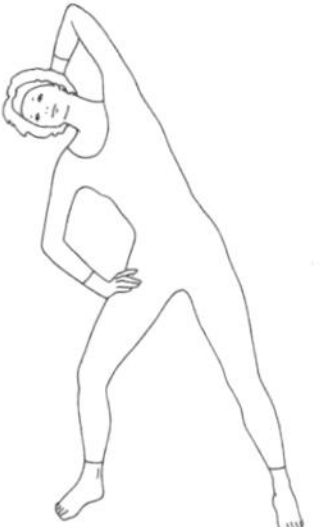

Standing lateral stretch (obliques and torso)

STRETCH #49

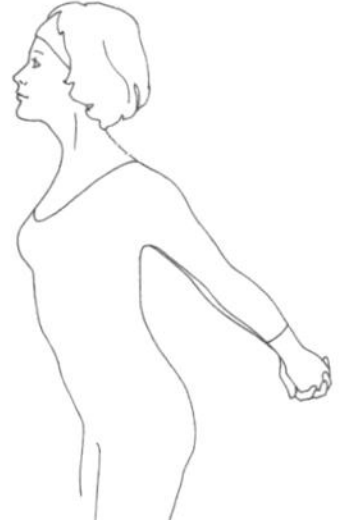

Arms low (chest)

STRETCH #58

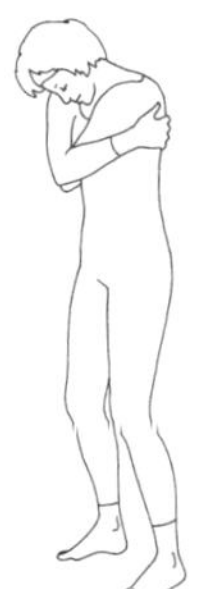

Hug yourself (upper back)

STRETCH #52

SEATED STRETCHES

Sitting takes a big toll on your body! It tightens your back, hips, legs, and buttocks and throws your neck, chest, and shoulders into a perpetual slump.

The best remedy for sitting all day is to get up and move as often as you can. Take the wheels off your desk chair; park in the furthest parking space; hide the remote control. When your body needs to move it sends these signals: your back aches, your energy plummets, and your brain feels drained. So stretch! Even if you're trapped in your seat (on a long flight, for instance) stretch in your chair.

Hands behind your head (chest and front of shoulders)

STRETCH #57

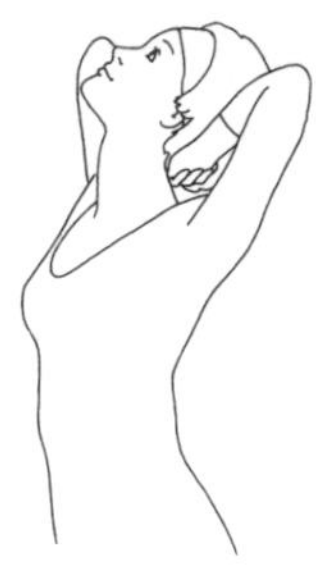

Overhead stretch (obliques and torso)

STRETCH #48

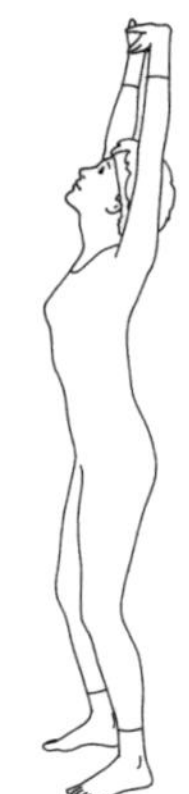

Lateral neck stretch

STRETCH #67

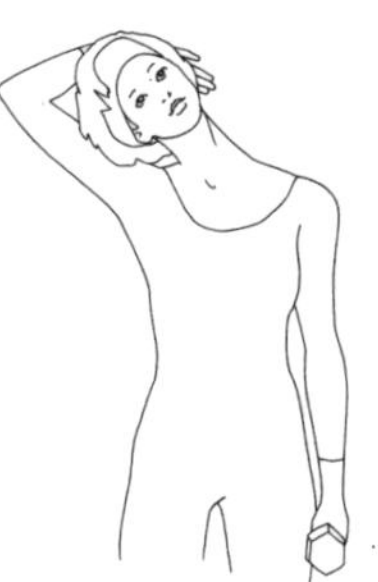

Oblique extensor stretch (neck)

STRETCH #68

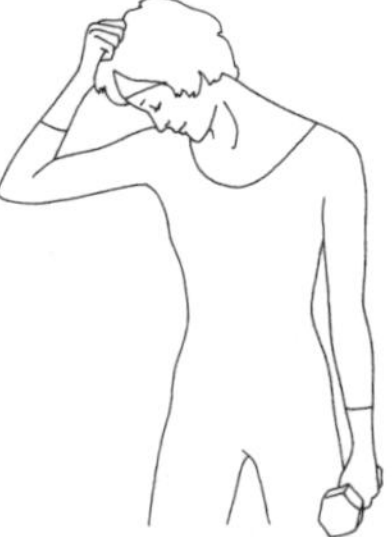

Seated lower-back stretch
STRETCH #3

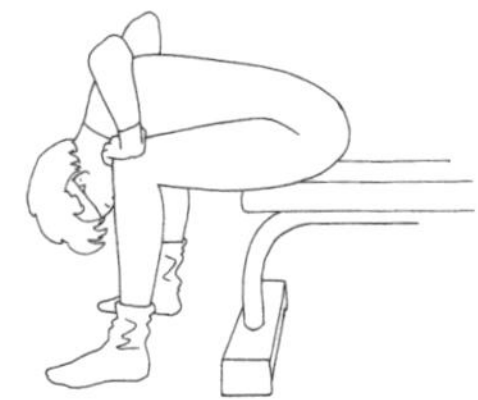

Seated or standing twist (lower back)
STRETCH #4

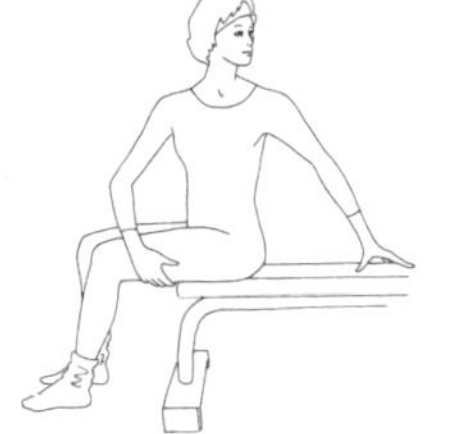

Seated hamstring stretch
STRETCH #28

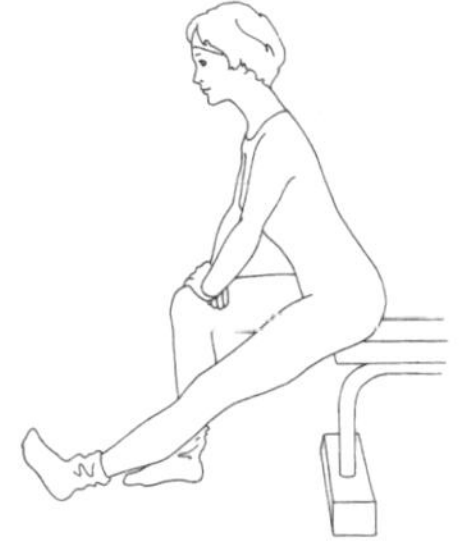

IF YOU STAND ALL DAY

If you have a job like cutting hair or working a cash register where you stand all day but don't move around much, you might get backaches and feel sluggish or light-headed. Standing still is tough on your lower back and legs because these muscles work hard to hold you upright. It also slows your circulation, since gravity pools the blood in your legs and feet. This means that lactic acid and other waste products don't get flushed from your legs, which can cause swollen ankles and feet. Moving and stretching can prevent all this.

It's also important to wear comfortable shoes that keep your spine in healthy alignment while you're standing on the job. Don't wear high heels—they put your lower back into an exaggerated arch (and shorten your calves and Achilles tendons). For extra relief, stand with one foot on a block (about six to ten inches high). Be sure to alternate feet and take as many mini stretch breaks as you can.

When you get home from work, lie on the floor with your legs resting up against a wall to reverse the blood flow in your legs.

Standing pelvic tilt (lower back)
STRETCH #8

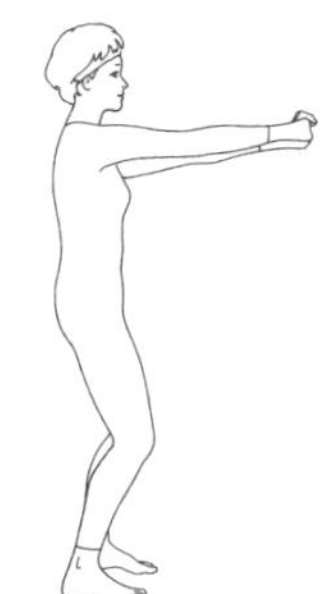

More advanced standing pelvic tilt (lower back)
STRETCH #9

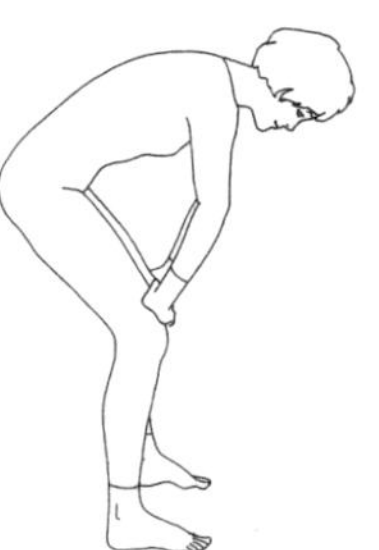

Sit-back stretch (upper back)
STRETCH #55

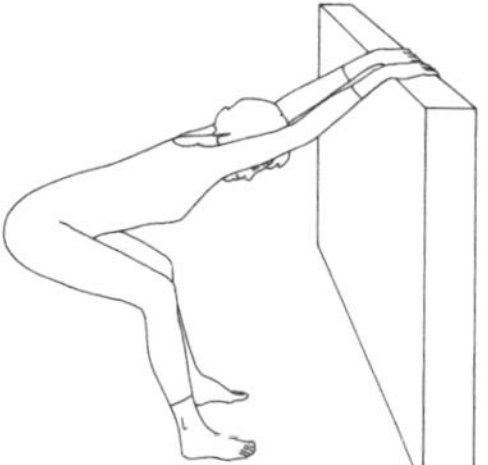

Foot-on-a-step stretch (hip flexors)
STRETCH #26

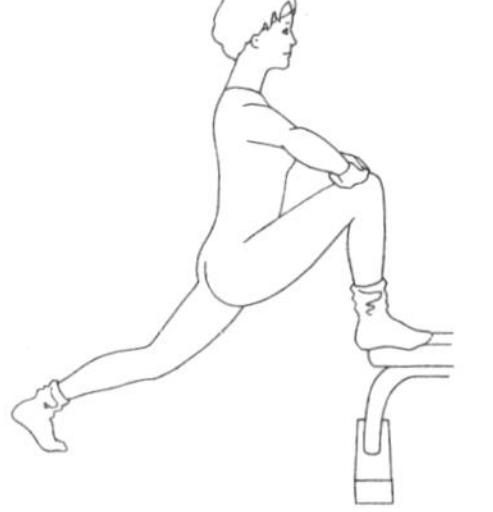

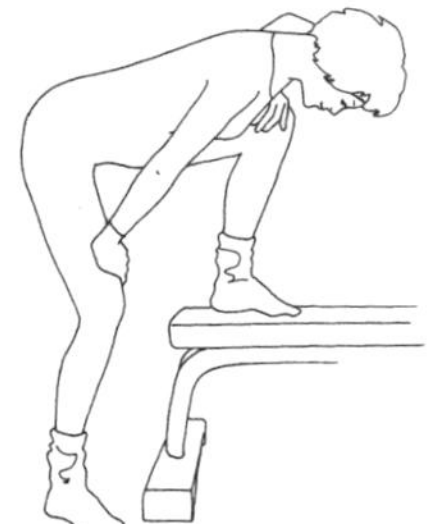

Hang over a chair (inner thigh)
STRETCH #36

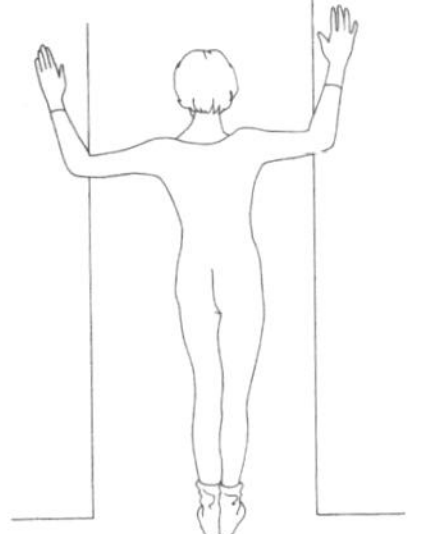

Doorway stretch (chest)
STRETCH #59

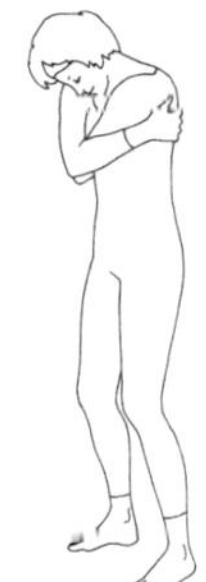

Hug yourself (upper back)
STRETCH #52

And when you get the chance to lie down, rest with your feet and legs lifted up against a wall and try:

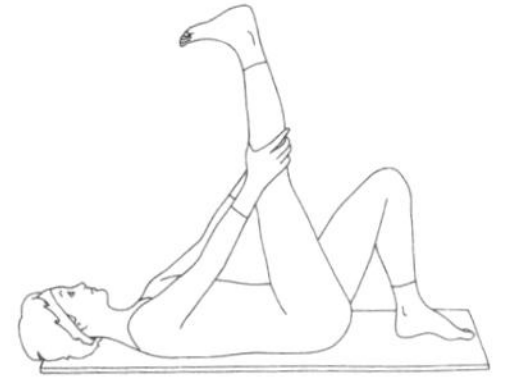

Leg-up hamstring stretch
STRETCH #27

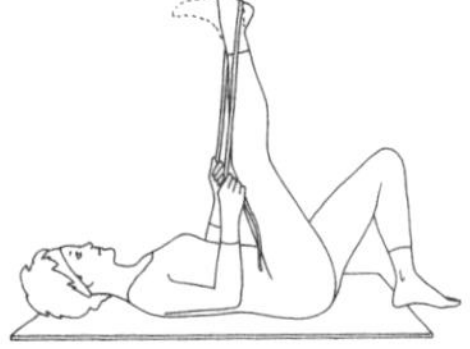

Flex and point (ankles and feet)
STRETCH #73

IF YOU LIFT, PUSH, AND PULL ALL DAY

You might think that a physically demanding job such as hauling, doing construction, or chasing toddlers would keep you fit. Heavy labor *can* be a workout, but most of the time it's not a balanced one. It tends to overwork the chest, shoulders, and triceps (the muscles that help you push, hammer, and hold things) and the back, shoulders, and biceps (the muscles that help you pull). Meanwhile, the core stabilizing muscles in the abdominals, lower back, and hips, as well as the little muscles in the wrists, ankles, elbows, and knees, become the weak links in the chain. These are the first things that give out.

Lifting heavy loads tightens muscles. Over time, unless you stretch, these tight muscles take more effort to move and you lose speed and coordination (which can make you more prone to accidents). Although few people do this, the best way to prepare the body for physically demanding labor is to get in shape and stay in shape—away from the job site. Create balanced muscle strength with a full weight-training routine, especially for the weak spots. Add aerobic exercise for endurance; stretch as often as you can and use pulleys and other leverage advantages to help lift heavy loads.

Erector spinae stretch (lower back)
STRETCH #2

Full-body stretch (abdominals)
STRETCH #45

One knee to chest (buttocks, hips, and lower back)
STRETCH #12

Knee across the body (buttocks, hips, and lower back)
STRETCH #13

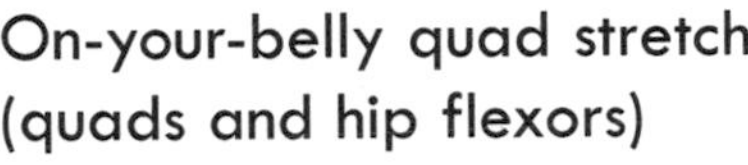

On-your-belly quad stretch (quads and hip flexors)
STRETCH #18

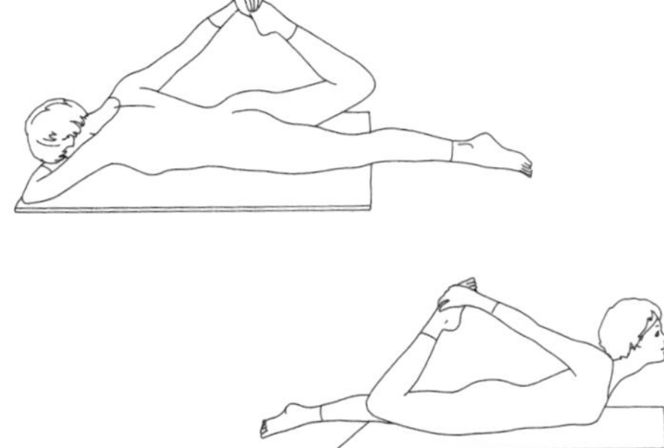

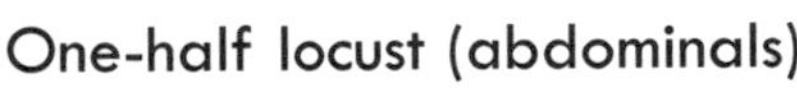

One-half locust (abdominals)
STRETCH #47

Floor or bench hamstring stretch
STRETCH #29

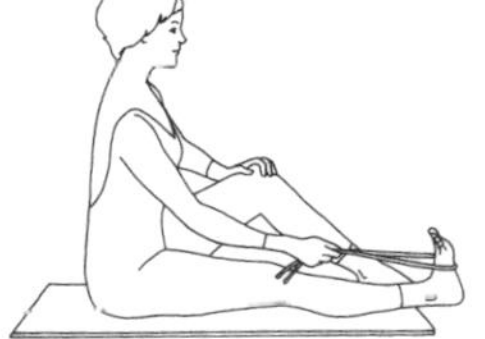

Posterior shoulder stretch
STRETCH #61

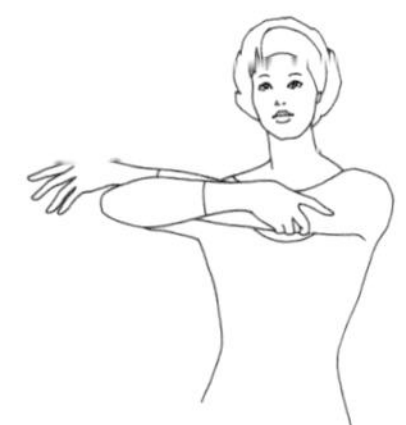

Arms low (chest)
STRETCH #58

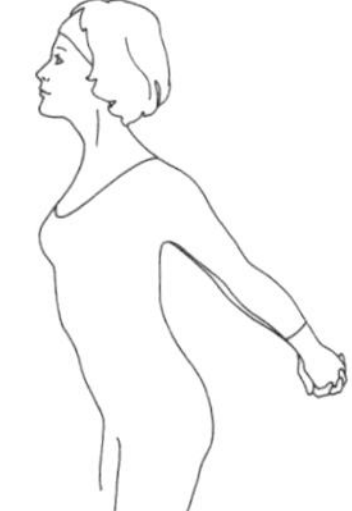

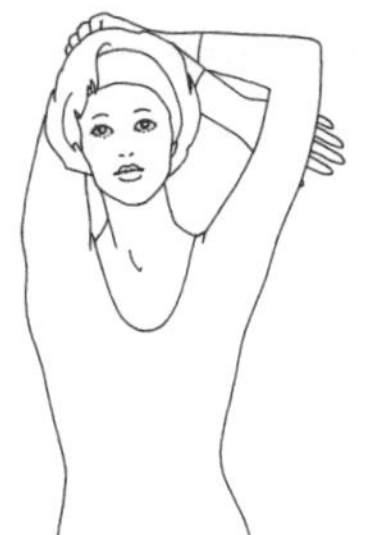

Triceps stretch (arms)
STRETCH #64

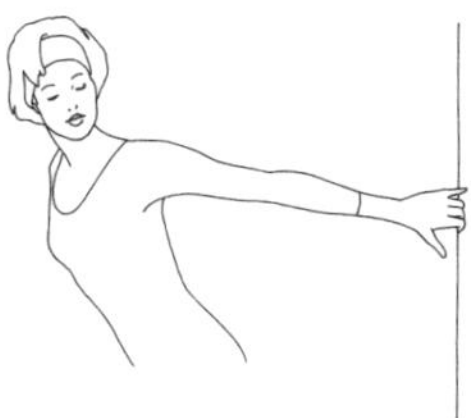

Biceps stretch (arms)
STRETCH #65

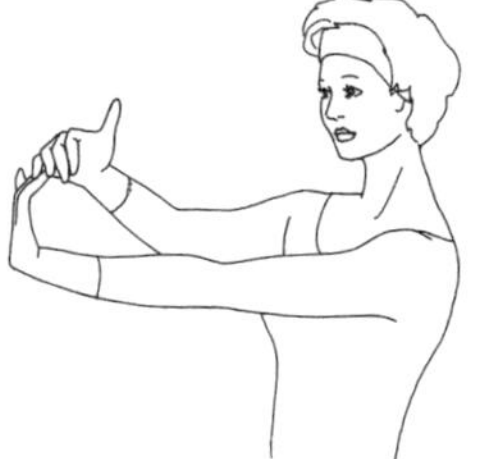

Wrist flexor stretch
STRETCH #69

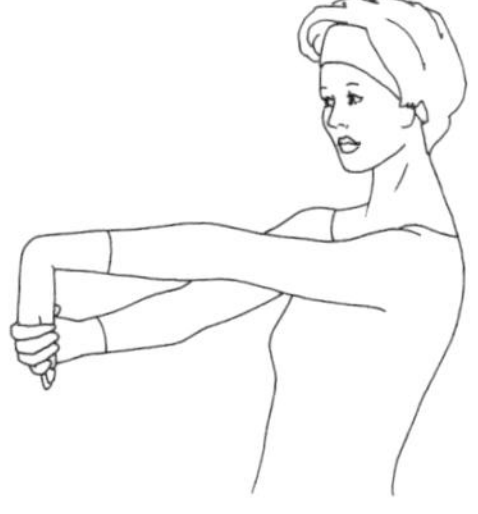

Wrist extensor stretch
STRETCH #70

NIGHTTIME STRETCHES

Doing vigorous exercise before going to bed can rev up your metabolism and keep you awake. A *gentle* stretching routine, however, can be very relaxing and help put you to sleep. Be sure to breathe slowly and deeply while you stretch. Hold each stretch for 30 seconds and move in a relaxed and easy manner from stretch to stretch.

Hug knees to chest (lower back)
STRETCH #1

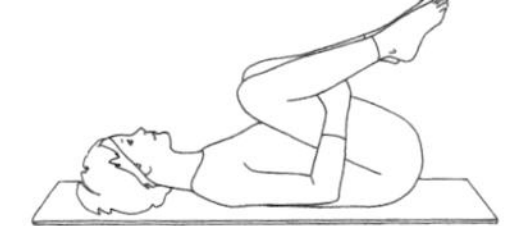

Erector spinae stretch (lower back)
STRETCH #2

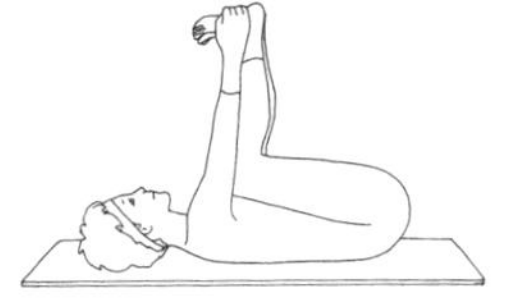

Leg-up hamstring stretch
STRETCH #27

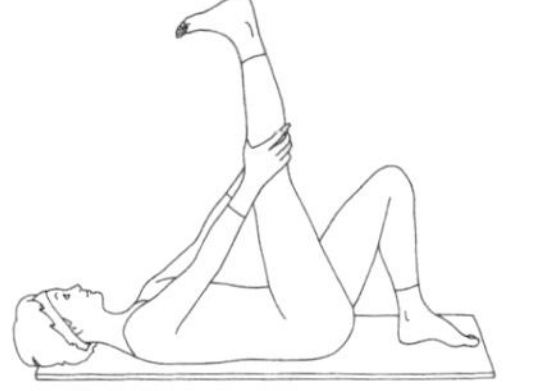

Pelvic tilt into bridge (lower back)
STRETCH #7

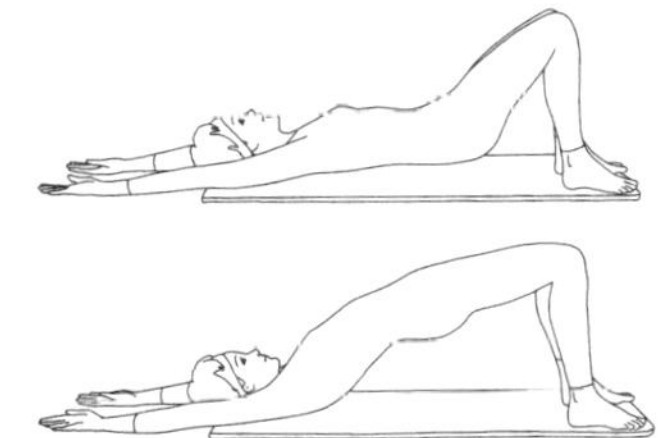

Knee across the body (buttocks, hips, and lower back)
STRETCH #13

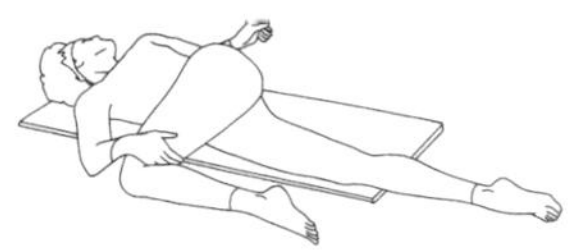

Ankle on the knee (buttocks, hips, and lower back)
STRETCH #14

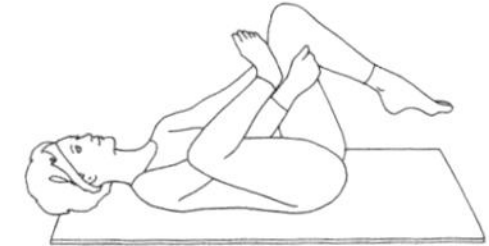

On-your-side quad stretch (quads and hip flexors)
STRETCH #19

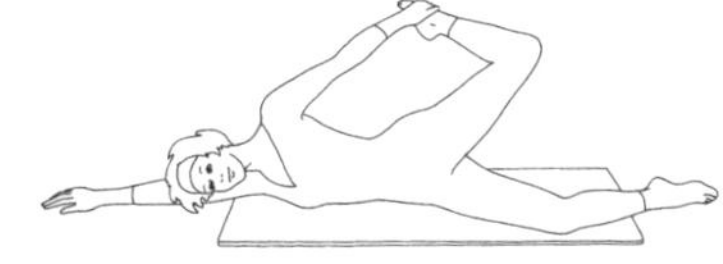

Cat stretch (lower back)
STRETCH #5

Child's pose (lower back)
STRETCH #6

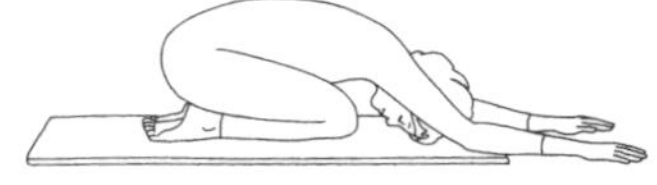

IF YOU'RE OVER FIFTY

Pictures of eighty- and ninety-year-old yogis holding pretzel postures and lotus positions attest to the mobility-enhancing power of stretching. You don't, however, have to be able to fold yourself into a pretzel to benefit from stretching. Even just 10 minutes a day of gentle stretching, plus regular walks and strength training twice a week, can make a huge impact on your well-being—and keep you fit and vital throughout your life! If you're over fifty and not used to following an exercise routine and you worry about when to integrate it into your life, do it first thing in the morning. Early-morning exercisers tend to stick with a program. Plus, once you do it, you can feel virtuous for the rest of the day.

As you embark on your stretches, don't force your body into uncomfortable positions or worry about how flexible you think you *should* be. Respect your body's twinges and avoid any positions that cause sharp pain. But don't baby yourself too much either or use the excuse that you're too old to challenge yourself or improve. If you're diligent and stretch regularly, your flexibility *will* improve—and this can give you a more robust posture and a more youthful appearance and will increase your energy and overall health.

One knee to chest (buttocks, hips, and lower back)
STRETCH #12

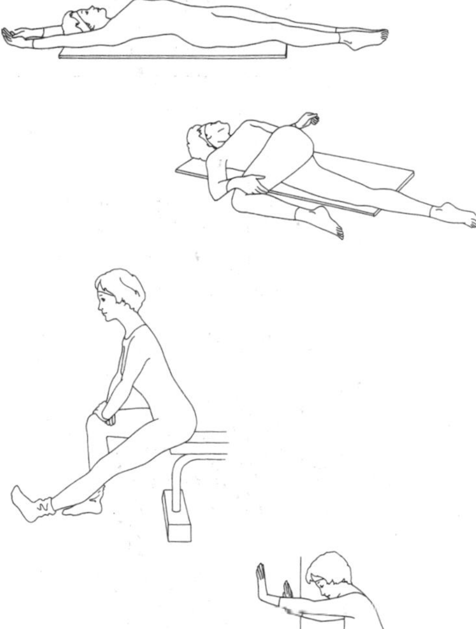

Full-body stretch (abdominals)
STRETCH #45

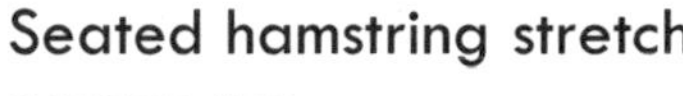

Knee across the body (buttocks, hips, and lower back)
STRETCH #13

Seated hamstring stretch
STRETCH #28

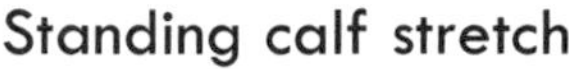

Standing calf stretch
STRETCH #39

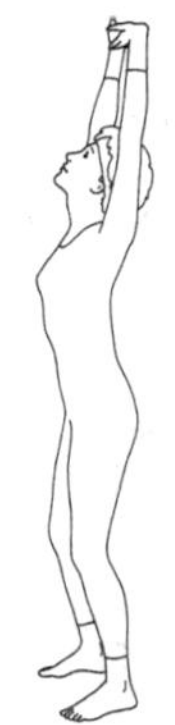

Overhead stretch (obliques and torso)
STRETCH #48

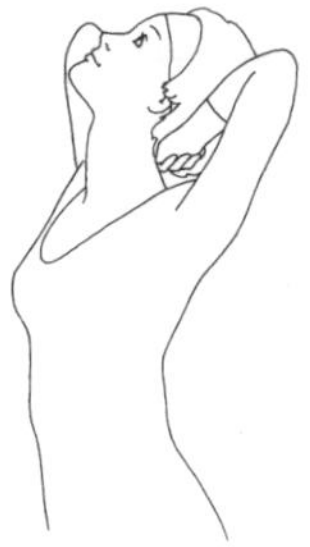

Hands behind your head (chest and front of shoulders)

STRETCH #57

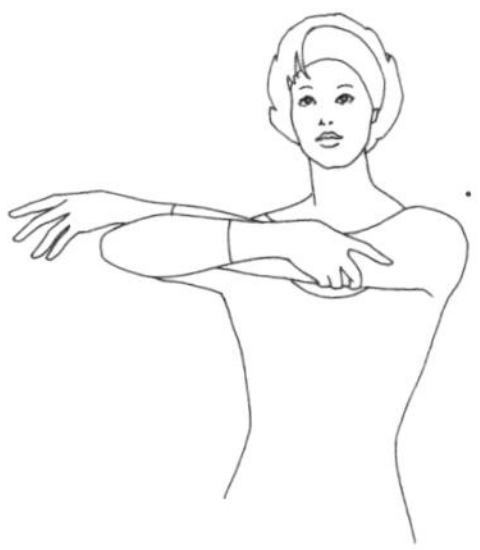

Posterior shoulder stretch

STRETCH #61

STRETCHES FOR SPORT AND FITNESS

AEROBIC DANCE

Whether you do high- or low-impact, step, hip-hop, or "flow" aerobic dance, your knees, hips, feet, and back can still take a beating, especially if you jump, dance on a concrete floor, have worn-out, nonsupportive shoes, or use bad form.

Well-trained, certified instructors typically include gentle stretches in a warm-up, followed by deeper stretches at the end of class. But you can't always count on that. So always be sure to stretch *after* class to stay flexible and prevent hip, knee, and back pain. Stretches #1–#7 are good to do after a 5-minute warm-up. Stretches #8–#14 work best at the end of a workout.

More advanced standing pelvic tilt (lower back)

STRETCH #9

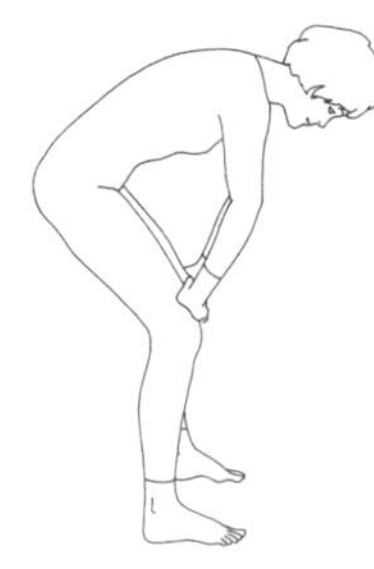

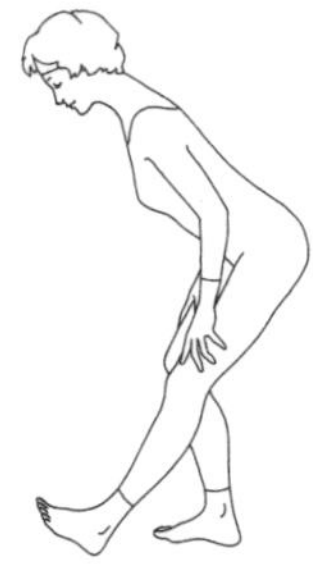

Standing hamstring stretch
STRETCH #30

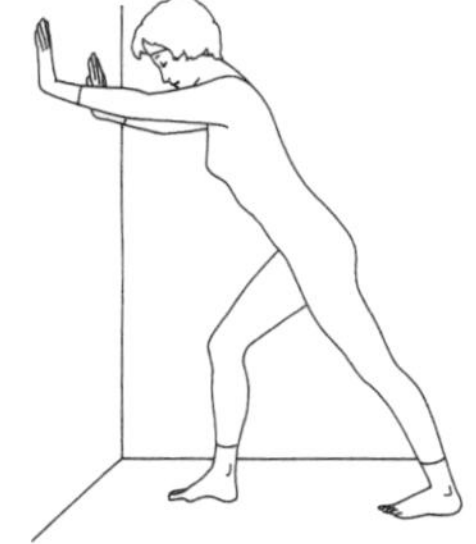

Standing calf stretch
STRETCH #39

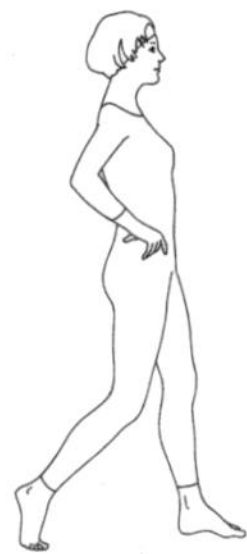

Standing hip flexor
STRETCH #23

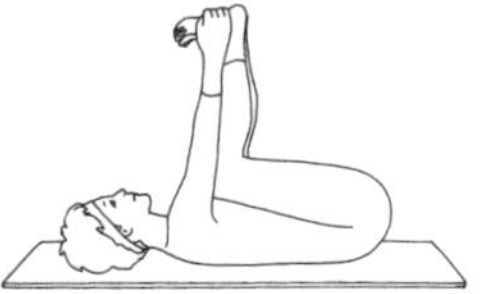

Erector spinae stretch (lower back)
STRETCH #2

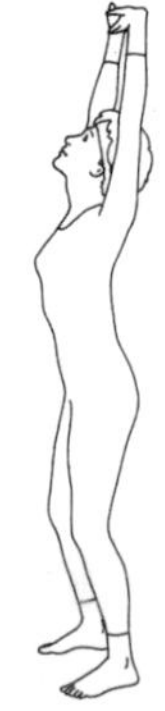

Overhead stretch (obliques and torso)
STRETCH #48

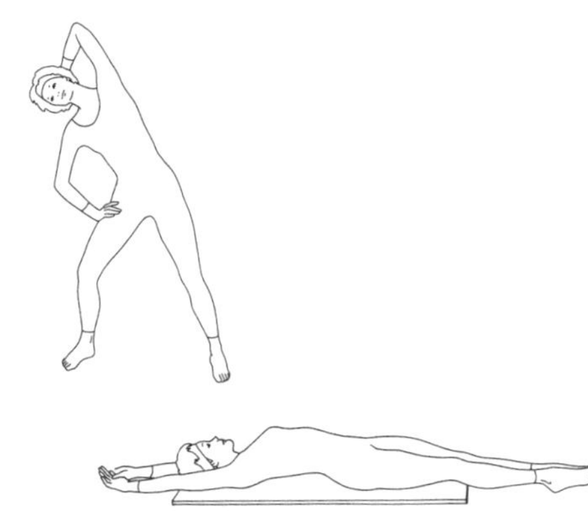

Standing lateral stretch (obliques and torso)
STRETCH #49

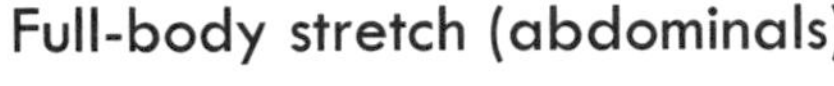

Full-body stretch (abdominals)
STRETCH #45

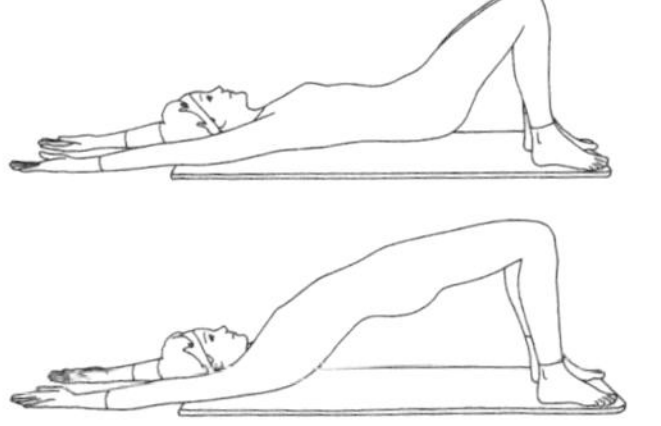

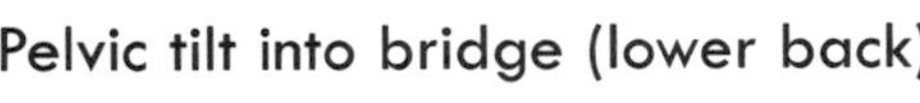

Pelvic tilt into bridge (lower back)
STRETCH #7

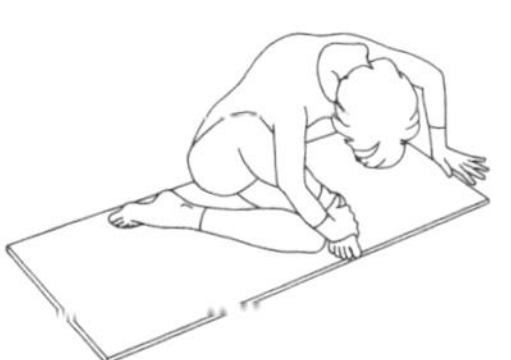

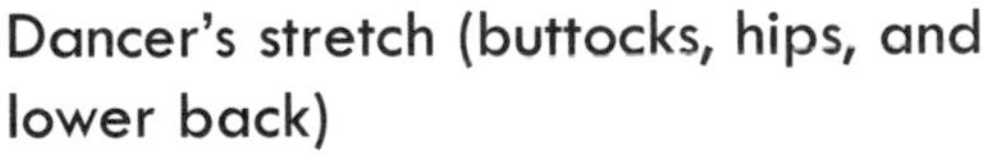

Dancer's stretch (buttocks, hips, and lower back)
STRETCH #16

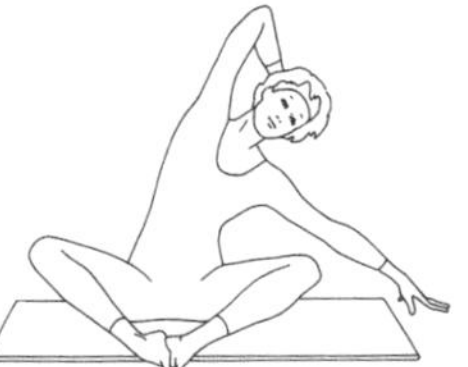

Seated overhead stretch (obliques and torso)
STRETCH #50

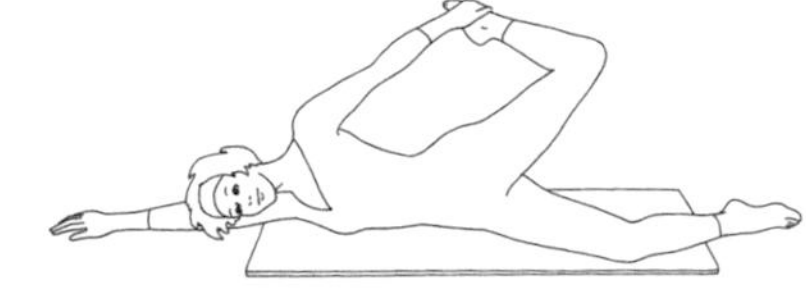

On-your-side quad stretch
STRETCH #19

Side-lying groin stretch (inner thigh)
STRETCH #35

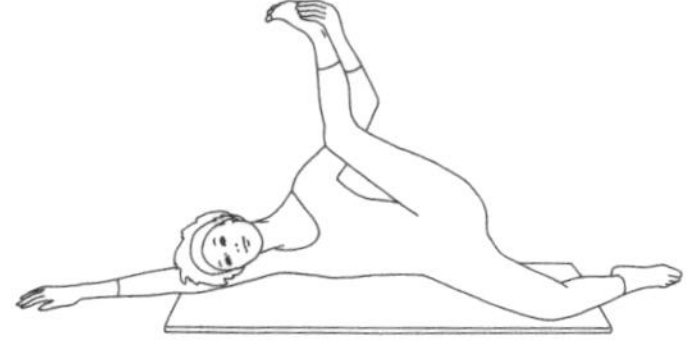

All-fours twist (upper back)
STRETCH #54

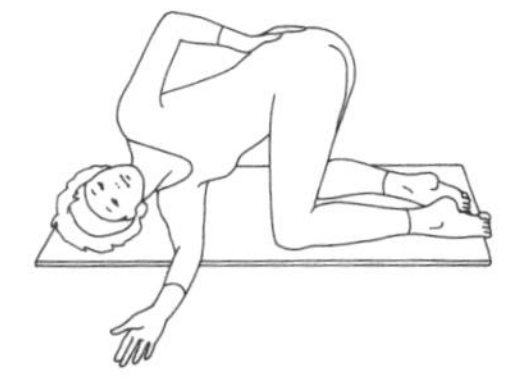

BASKETBALL

Basketball is a high-risk game. It's nonstop and full of sudden and repetitive moves. Every jump shot brings you back to earth with several times your body weight; plus, you can easily run right smack into another player—so it isn't difficult to get hurt. At highest risk are the tendons, ligaments, and muscles that stabilize your joints, especially around the knees, ankles, lower back, hips, and shoulders. A full-body stretching routine—including stretches for the little muscles in the wrists and ankles—won't prevent all injuries, but it can help keep your reflexes sharp and speed the recovery time if you do get injured.

Today, many coaches, aware of the importance of flexibility, send their players to yoga and stretch classes as often as they send them to the gym. These stretches work well after a game, on days off, as well as in the off-season.

Overhead stretch (obliques and torso)
STRETCH #48

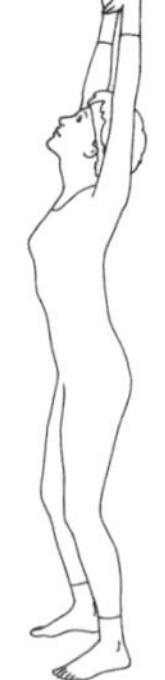

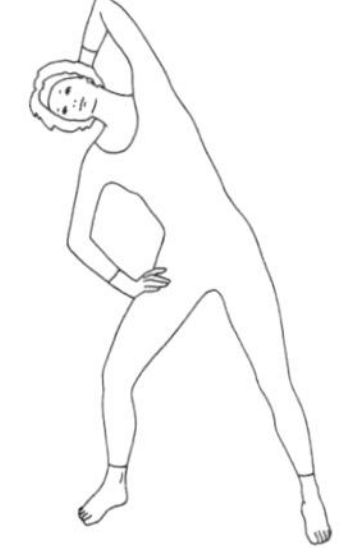

Standing lateral stretch (obliques and torso)
STRETCH #49

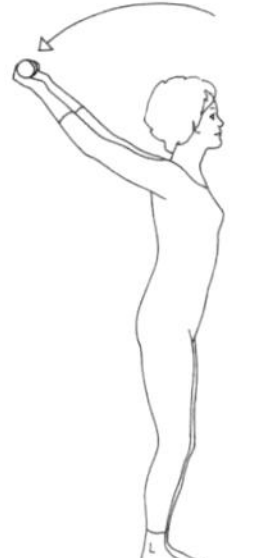

Chest and front-of-shoulder stretch (pole)
STRETCH #81

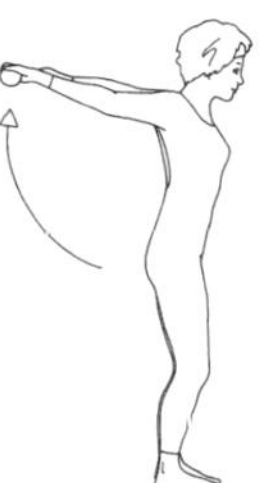

Round-the-world shoulder stretch (pole)
STRETCH #82

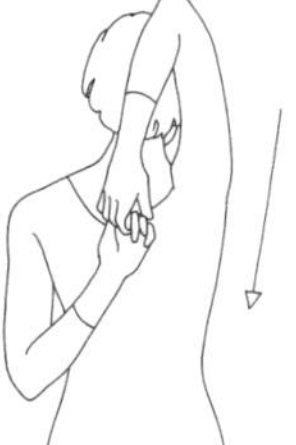

External rotator stretch (shoulders and arms)
STRETCH #62

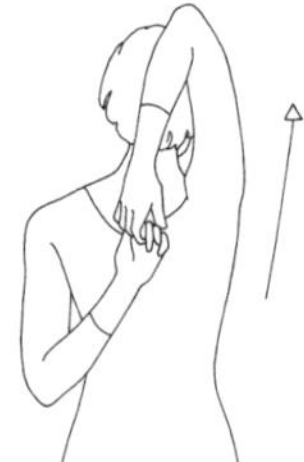

Internal rotator stretch (shoulders and arms)
STRETCH #63

Hug yourself (upper back)
STRETCH #52

Erector spinae stretch (lower back)
STRETCH #2

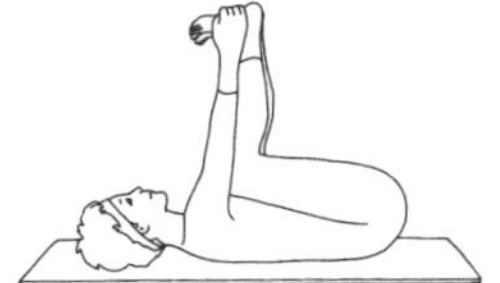

Knee across the body (buttocks, hips, and lower back)
STRETCH #13

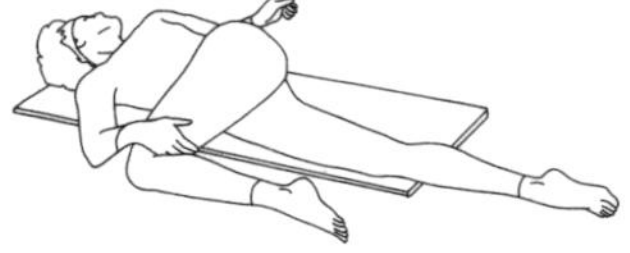

Ankle on the knee (buttocks, hips, and lower back)
STRETCH #14

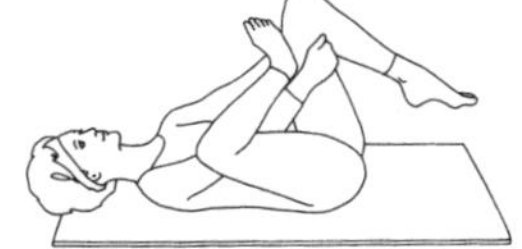

Back-of-the-neck stretch
STRETCH #66

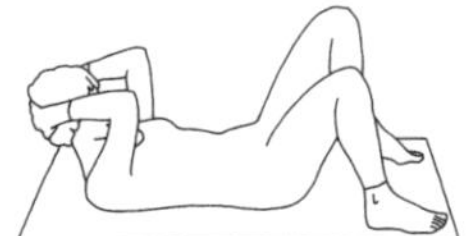

Standing hamstring stretch
STRETCH #30

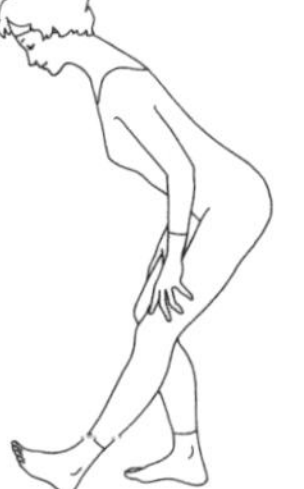

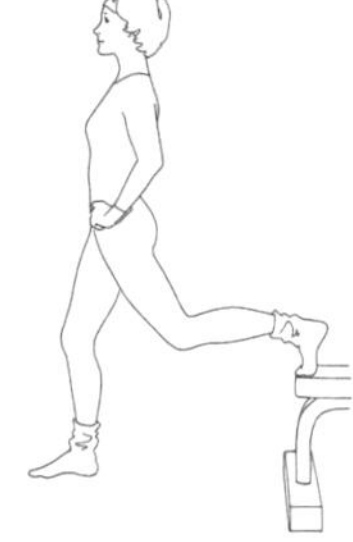

Standing elevated quad stretch (quads and hip flexors)

STRETCH #22

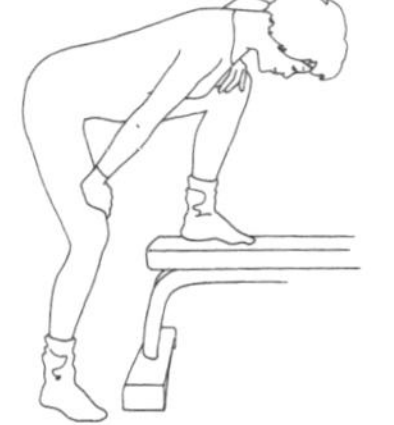

Hang over a chair (inner thigh)

STRETCH #36

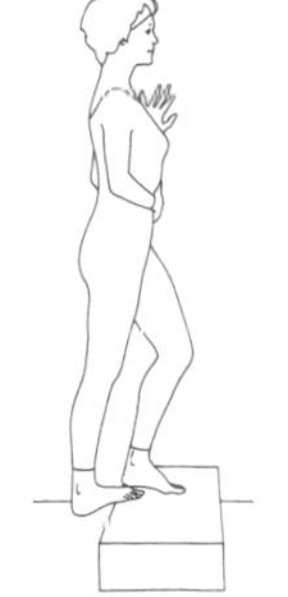

The stair stretch (calves and Achilles)

STRETCH #43

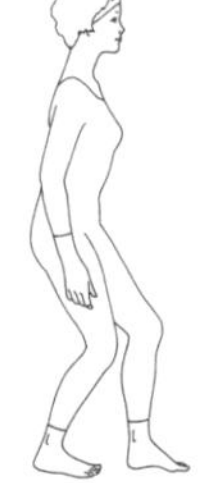

Standing soleus and Achilles stretch

STRETCH #42

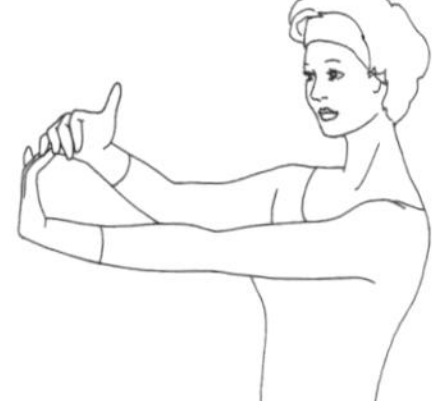

Wrist flexor stretch

STRETCH #69

Wrist extensor stretch
STRETCH #70

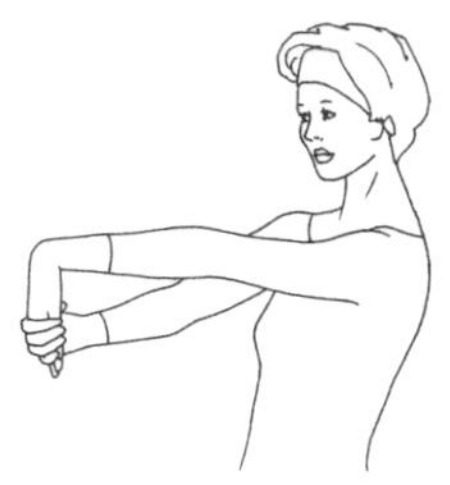

BICYCLING

Although bicycling is a nonimpact sport (unless you fall onto the pavement, of course), it can still make your muscles tight, so you have to stretch. Cycling is a mostly lower- and middle-body activity. Pressing the pedal down works the quads, hip extensors, and shin muscles. Pulling the pedal up uses the hips, hamstrings, and calves. If your body pitches forward over the handlebars, your abdominals, lower back, upper torso, and shoulders will also work to keep you stable.

Make sure to adjust your seat properly. If your seat is too low, you'll feel extra pressure on your knees and hips. If you ride bent over your handlebars for long periods of time, stand up on your pedals every once in a while or sit up straight to ease lower-back pain and shoulder strain. For balanced all-over strength, be sure to supplement your cycling with an upper-body strength-training routine.

Full-body stretch (abdominals)
STRETCH #45

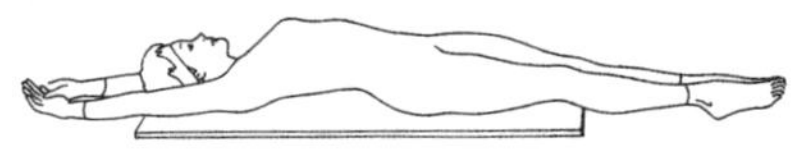

One knee to chest (buttocks, hips, and lower back)
STRETCH #12

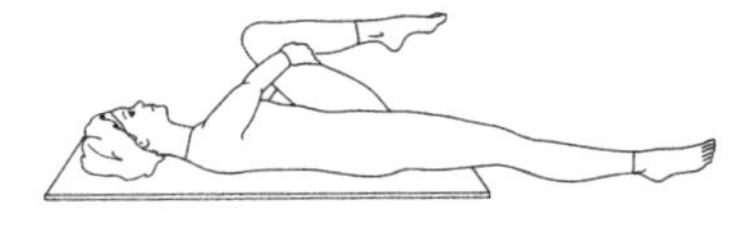

Knee across the body (buttocks, hips, and lower back)
STRETCH #13

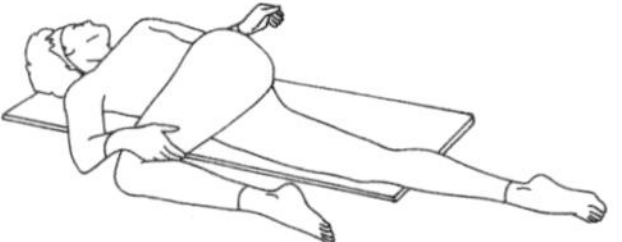

Ankle on the knee (buttocks, hips, and lower back)
STRETCH #14

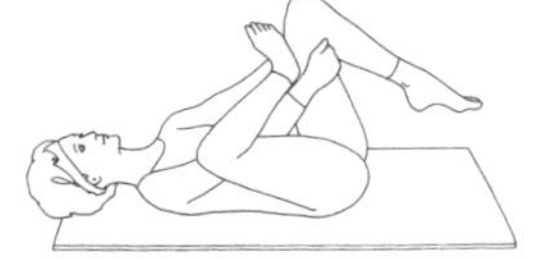

Cat stretch (lower back)
STRETCH #5

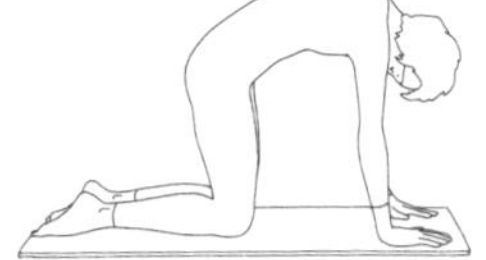

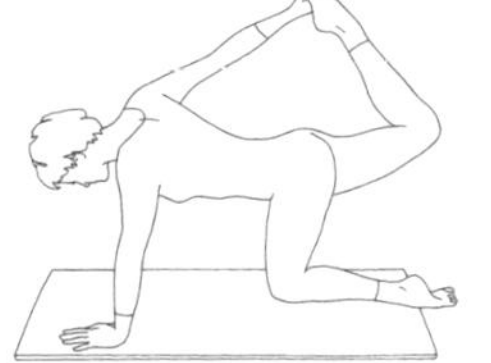

All-fours quad stretch
STRETCH #21

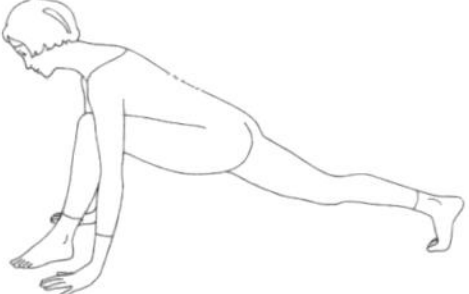

Runner's stretch (hip flexors)
STRETCH #25

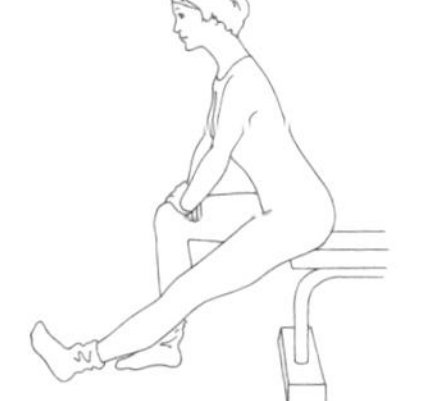

Seated hamstring stretch
STRETCH #28

Seated calf stretch
STRETCH #41

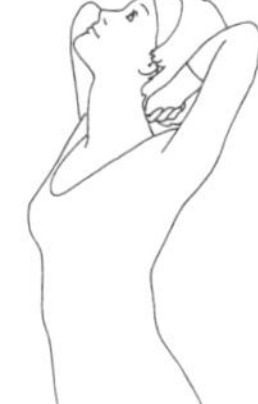

Hands behind your head (chest and front of shoulders)
STRETCH #57

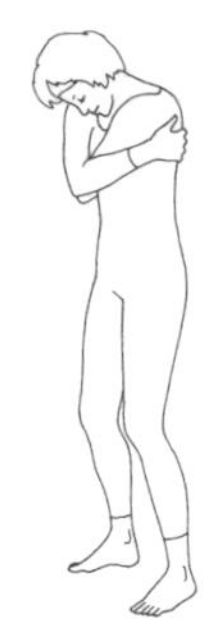

Hug yourself (upper back)
STRETCH #52

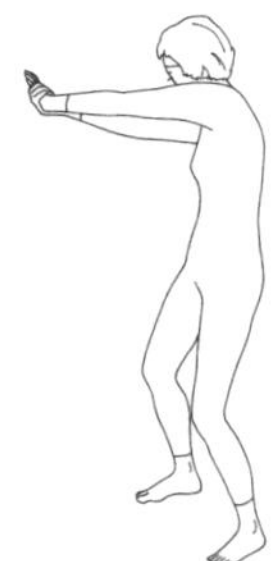

Side wrist pull (upper back)
STRETCH #53

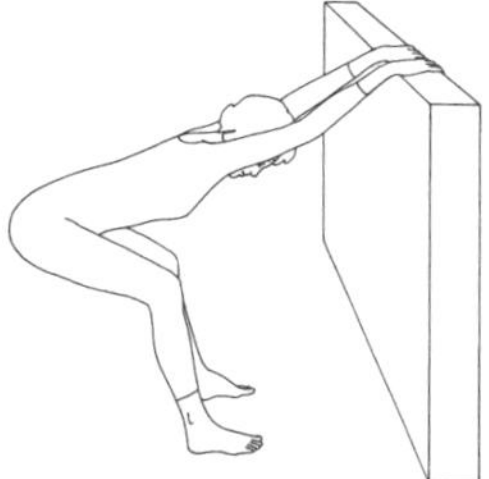

Sit-back stretch (upper back)
STRETCH #55

CLIMBING

Whether you scale a true rock face or a gym wall, climbing is a full-body activity that uses all the major muscles, as well as the tiniest muscles in the hands and feet. To pull yourself up a vertical wall, you need strength, flexibility, coordination, endurance, and the concentration to plan your next four moves. Chances are good you'll find yourself in some strange positions, hanging by just your fingers and toes. To prepare yourself for this, you'd better be relatively strong and flexible *before* you go up there. Be sure to plan ahead and hit the weights, do your aerobic exercise, and stretch.

Although you'll often stretch while you climb, we suggest that you gently stretch *before* you climb to prepare your body and mind; afterward, give yourself a deeper stretch so you won't become sore.

Erector spinae stretch (lower back)
STRETCH #2

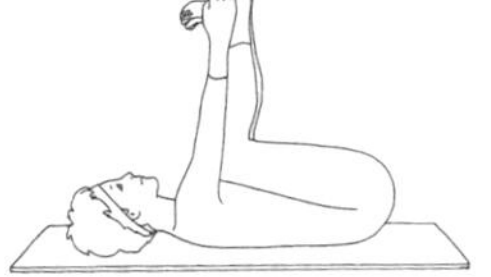

Pelvic tilt into bridge (lower back)
STRETCH #7

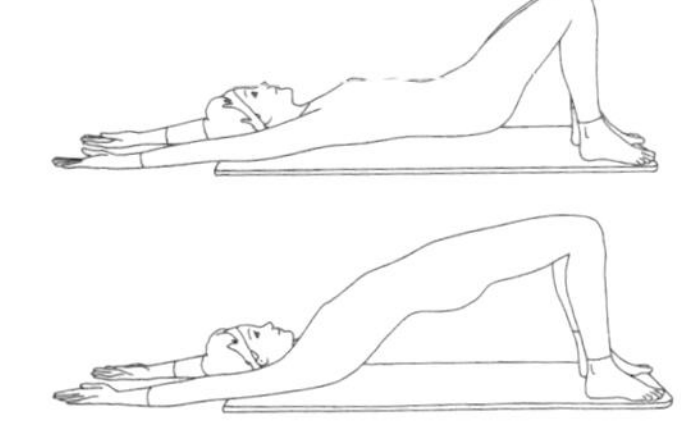

The full squat (lower back)
STRETCH #11

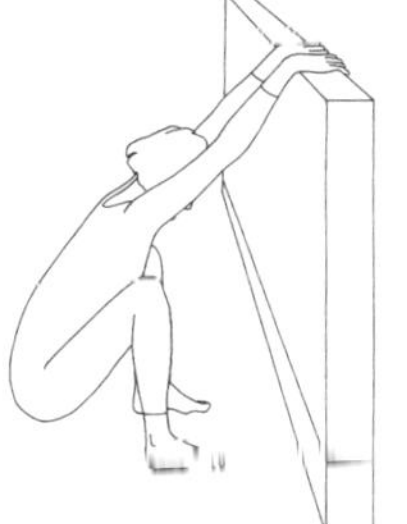

Seated floor twist (buttocks, hips, and lower back)
STRETCH #15

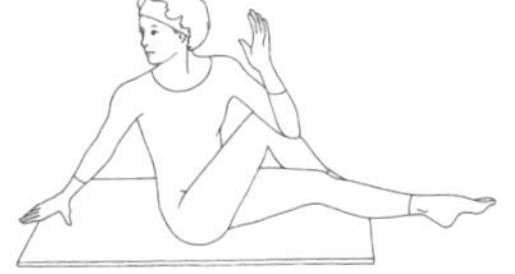

Toe grab and spread (ankles and feet)
STRETCH #74

Dancer's stretch (buttocks, hips, and lower back)
STRETCH #16

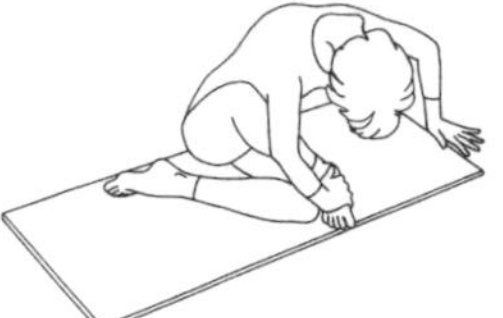

Bench hip flexor stretch
STRETCH #24

Side-lying stretch on a bench (outer hip and thigh)
STRETCH #32

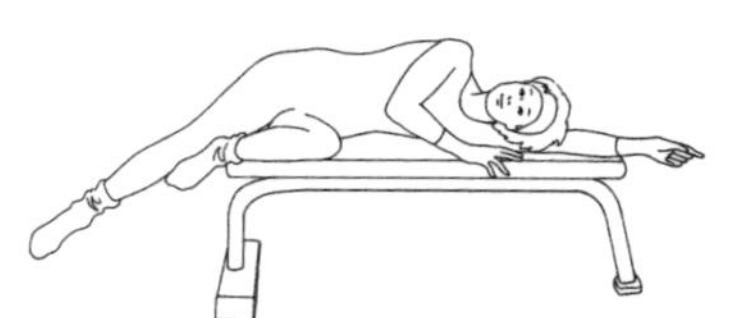

Standing elevated quad stretch
STRETCH #22

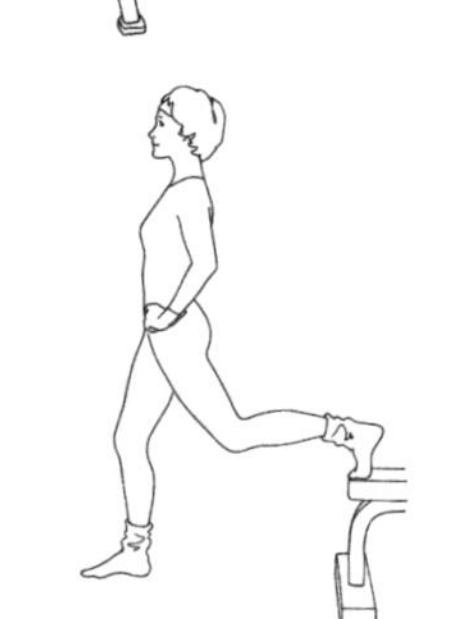

Foot-on-a-step stretch (hip flexors)
STRETCH #26

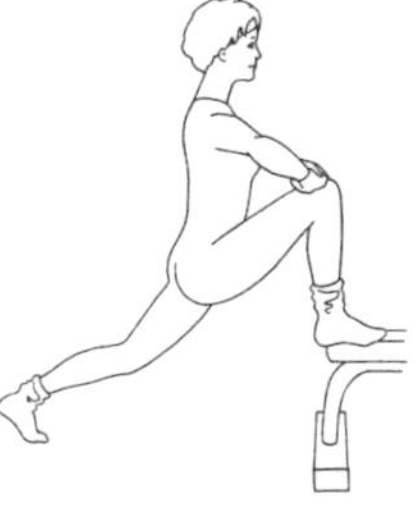

Standing inner-thigh stretch
STRETCH #37

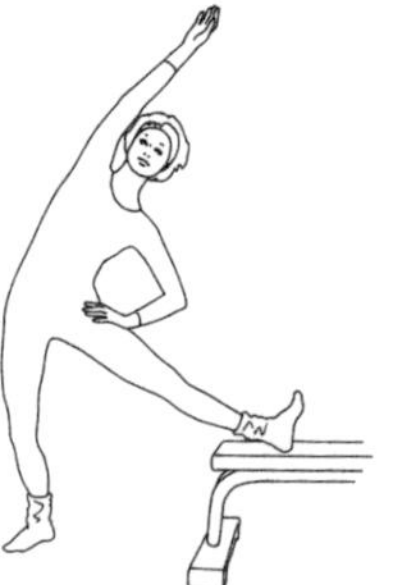

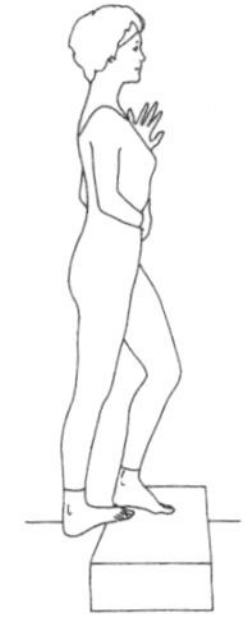

The stair stretch (calves and Achilles)
STRETCH #43

Starting-block Achilles stretch
STRETCH #44

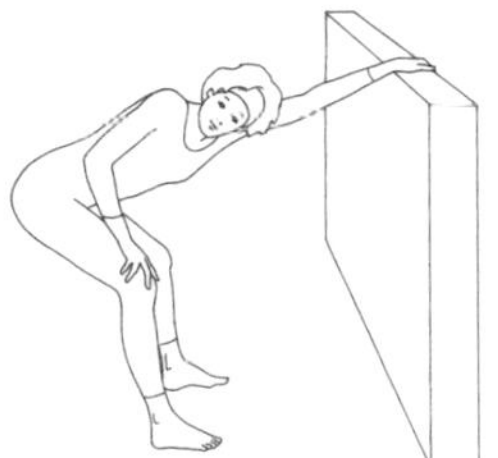

One-arm sit-back stretch (upper back)
STRETCH #56

On-your-knees chair stretch (chest and front of shoulders)
STRETCH #60

Posterior shoulder stretch
STRETCH #61

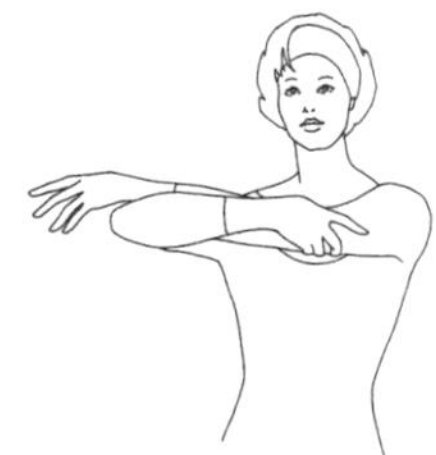

Triceps stretch (shoulders and arms)
STRETCH #64

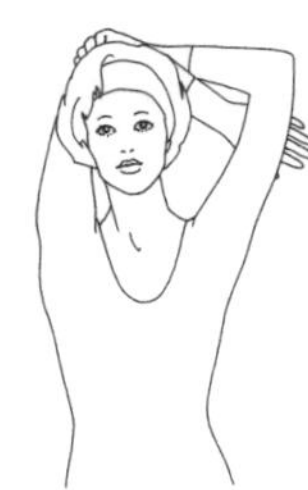

Biceps stretch (shoulders and arms)
STRETCH #65

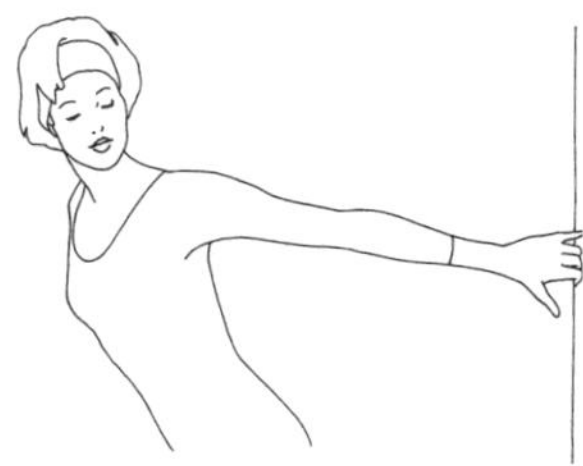

Wrist flexor stretch
STRETCH #69

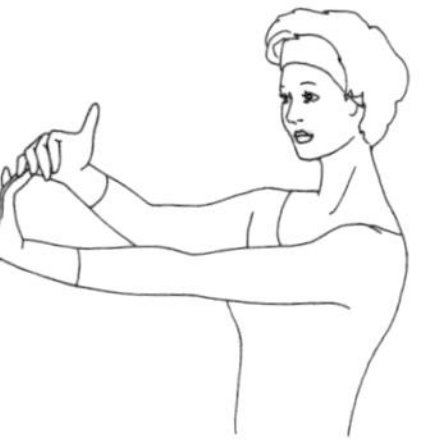

Wrist extensor stretch
STRETCH #70

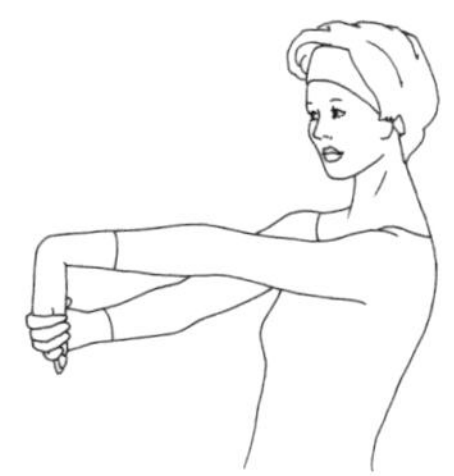

Finger stretches
STRETCH #72

DANCE AND GYMNASTICS

Dancers and gymnasts work hard to be superflexible but often take a good thing too far. In gymnastics, a sign of success is a dangerous swayback. In dance, it's the ability to kick your leg over your head. Although these things are impressive to watch, they can spell trouble. Supermobile joints are often held together by overstretched connective tissue, which can leave athletes vulnerable to injury and arthritis later in life. (About that swayback: some arching of the lower back is fine and healthy if the abdominal and lower-back muscles are strong enough to support it, but too much arching can lead to permanent disc damage and pain. As for kicking your leg over your head—some people just have more "turnout" than others do. This shouldn't determine a dancer's worth—particularly as he or she gets older!)

Young dancers and gymnasts often feel tremendous pressure to be ultrafit or thin. Excessive dieting combined with hard training (plus smoking and drinking sodas) can lead to premature osteoporosis. In order to be *healthy* but not obsessive, athletes, dancers, and gymnasts should eat more calories (of healthy food) more frequently than nonathletes, and they should supplement their dance and gymnastics with strength training, aerobic exercise, and a *sensible* flexibility routine (they shouldn't take stretches into the danger zone just because they can).

Gymnasts and dancers need the most strength work in the muscles surrounding their hips, knees, shoulders, and lower backs (where they're most often injured). They need the most flexibility in the groin, hamstrings, torso, feet, and calves.

In addition to the stretches below, dancers and gymnasts may also want to try the ball and water stretches.

Erector spinae stretch (lower back)

STRETCH #2

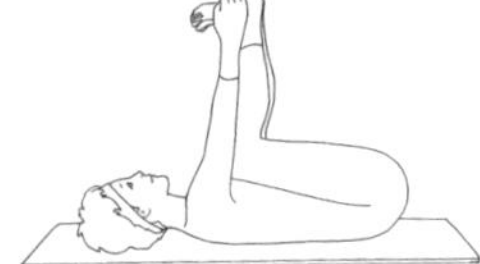

Pelvic tilt into bridge (lower back)
STRETCH #7

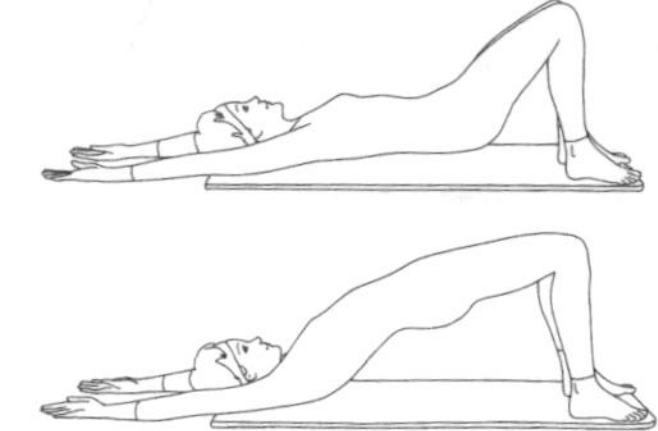

Leg-up hamstring stretch
STRETCH #27

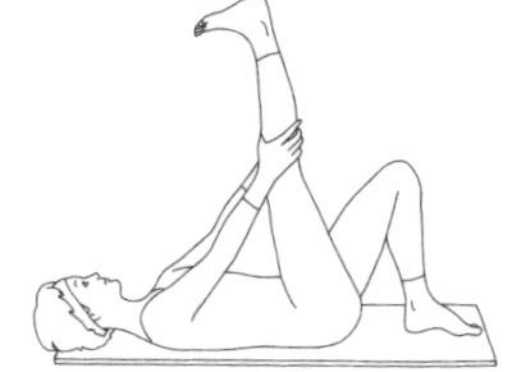

Toe grab and spread (ankles and feet)
STRETCH #74

On-your-side quad stretch
STRETCH #19

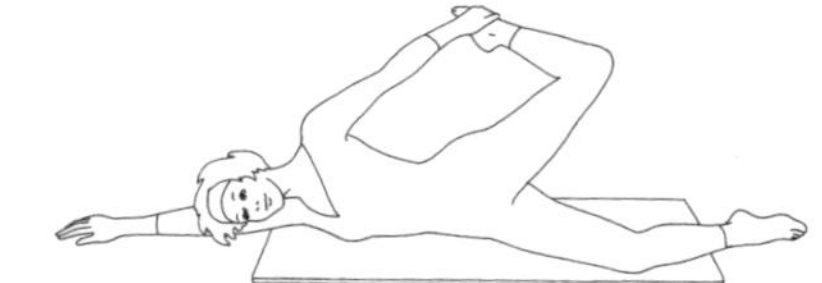

Side-lying floor stretch (outer hip and thigh)
STRETCH #31

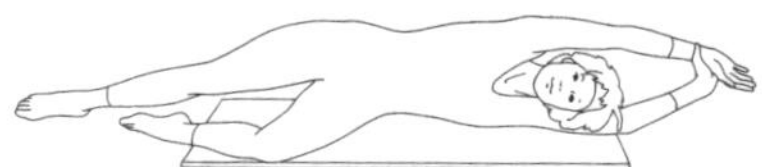

The straddle (inner thigh)
STRETCH #38

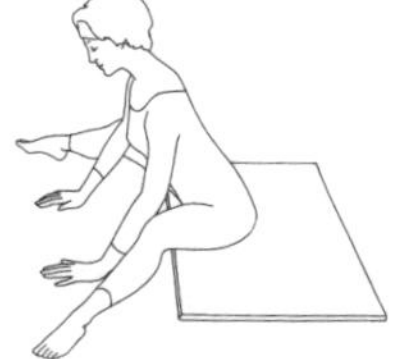

Dancer's stretch (buttocks, hips, and lower back)
STRETCH #16

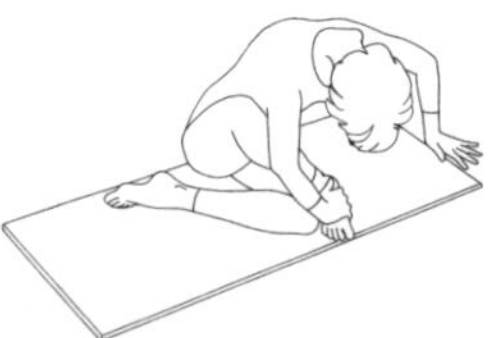

All-fours twist (upper back)
STRETCH #54

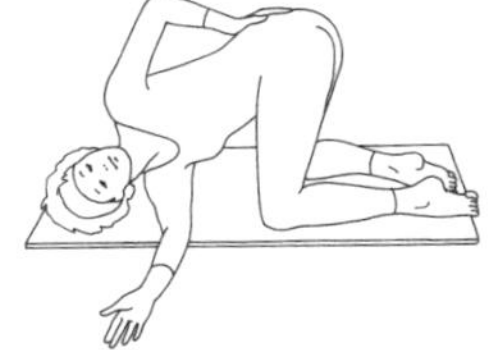

Overhead stretch (obliques and torso)
STRETCH #48

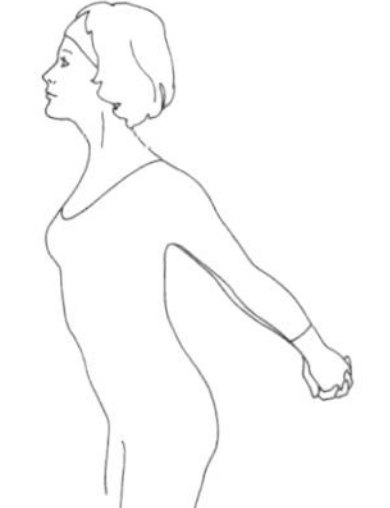

Arms low (chest)
STRETCH #58

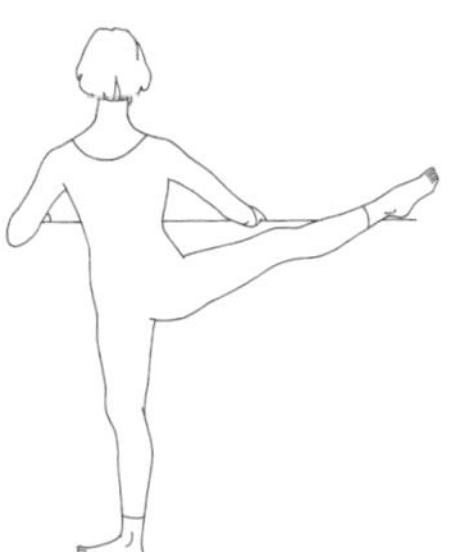

Inner-thigh stretch (ballet barre)
STRETCH #85

Inner-thigh and torso stretch (ballet barre)
STRETCH #86

Inner-thigh and opposite torso stretch (ballet barre)
STRETCH #87

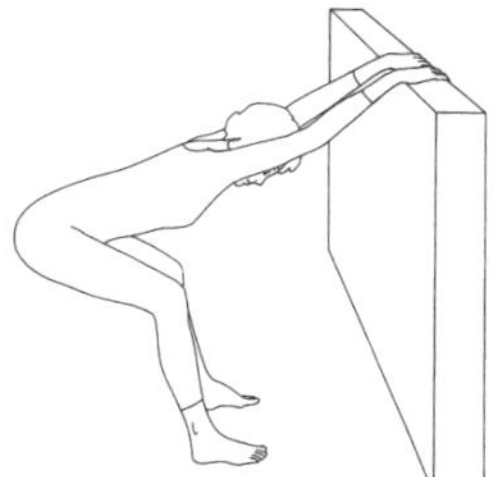

Sit-back stretch (upper back)
STRETCH #55

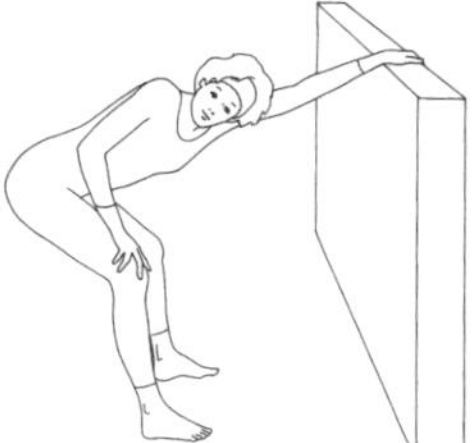

One-arm sit-back stretch (upper back)
STRETCH #56

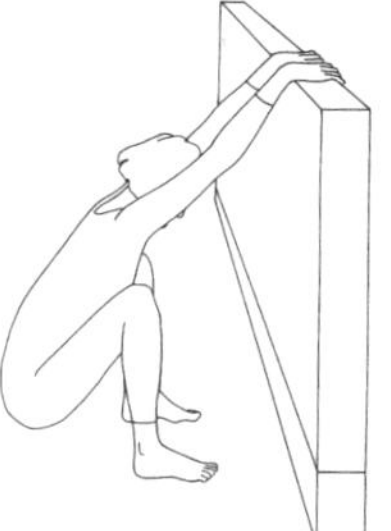

The full squat (lower back)
STRETCH #11

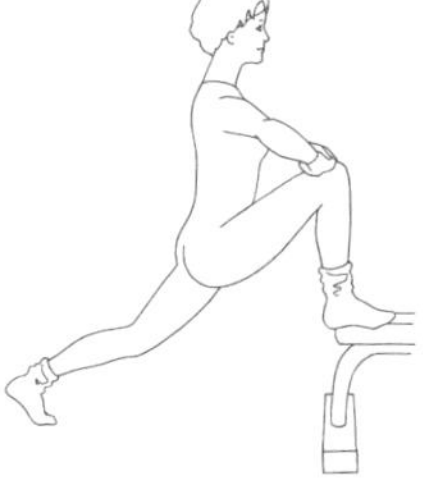

Foot-on-a-step stretch (hip flexors)
STRETCH #26

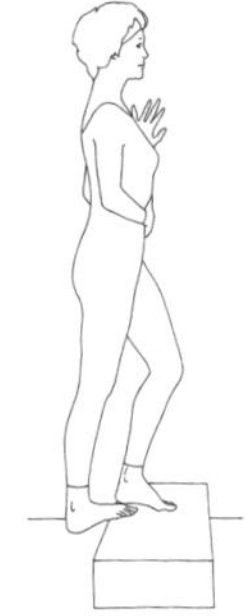

The stair stretch (calves and Achilles)
STRETCH #43

Starting-block Achilles stretch
STRETCH #44

GOLF

You might not think you need to be flexible to play golf. But if you want a decent golf swing, you need flexible hips, torso muscles, shoulders, arms, and wrists. These give your swing a bigger windup, so you hit the ball both harder and farther and have more control over where it goes.

Although in some circles it's not de rigueur to stretch on the links, it can be a good idea—and you can even use a golf club to help you do it. A few brief stretches before your game can help you relax, loosen up, and focus your mind. Stretching between holes can help ease the mounting mental frustration that often goes with the game; also, by then your muscles are warm and can stretch further. Stretching after you play or on your days off can permanently improve your flexibility.

Golf can be a legitimate workout by itself—but only if you walk the links. So skip the golf cart and, while you're at it, carry your own clubs.

Chest and front-of-shoulder stretch (pole)

STRETCH #81

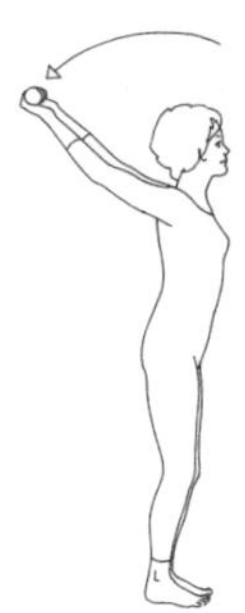

Round-the-world shoulder stretch (pole)

STRETCH #82

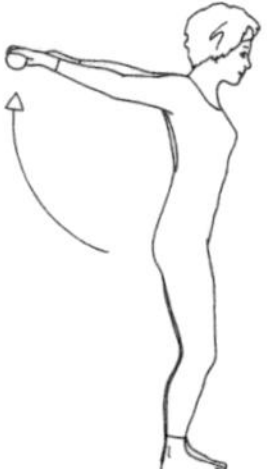

Side torso stretch (pole)

STRETCH #83

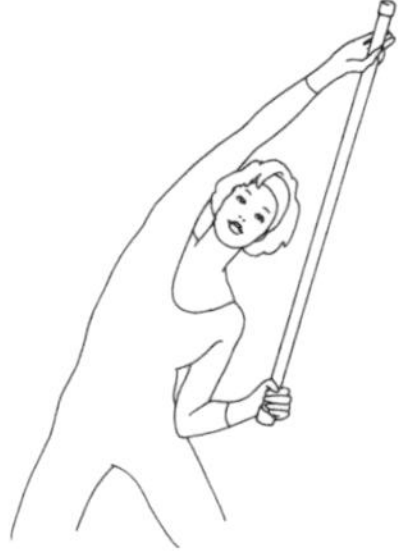

Hug a pole

STRETCH #84

Standing quad stretch

STRETCH #20

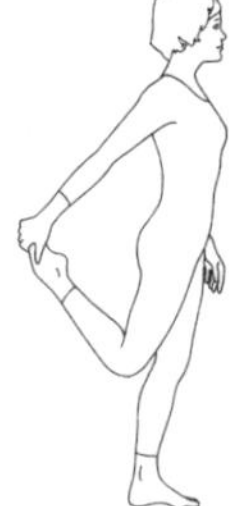

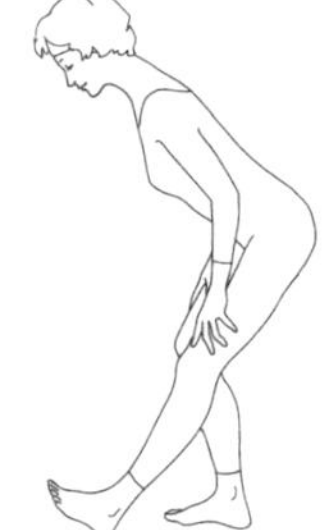

Standing hamstring stretch
STRETCH #30

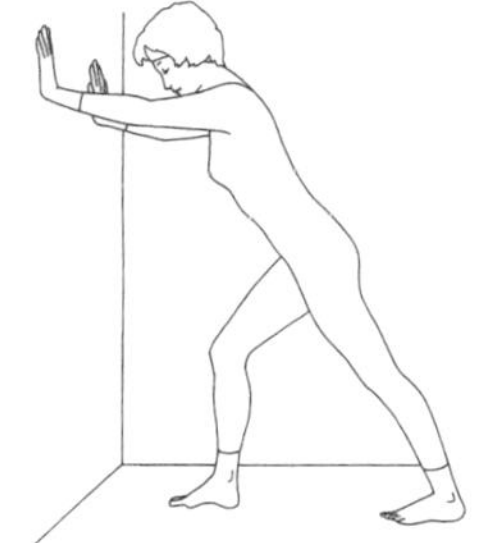

Standing calf stretch
STRETCH #39

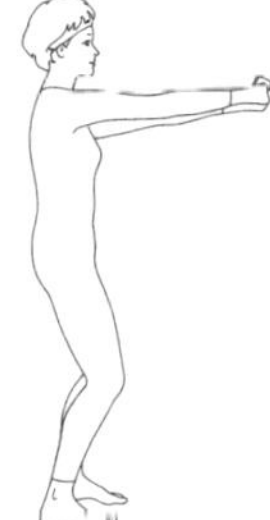

Standing pelvic tilt (lower back)
STRETCH #8

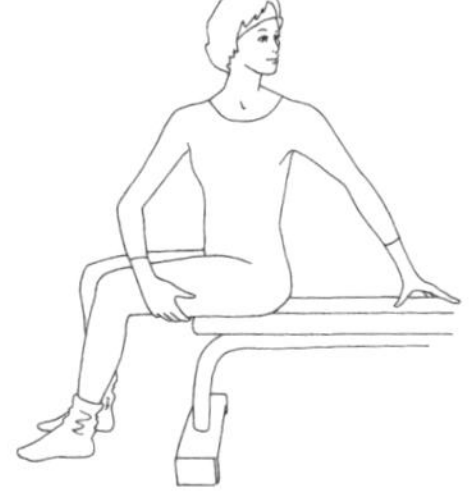

Seated or standing twist (lower back)
STRETCH #4

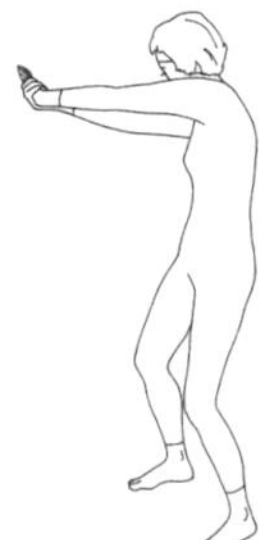

Side wrist pull (upper back)
STRETCH #53

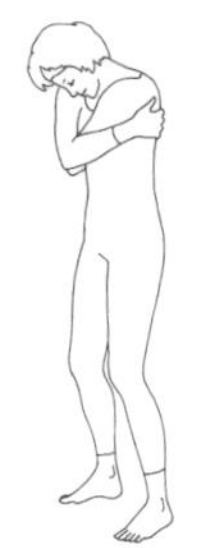

Hug yourself (upper back)
STRETCH #52

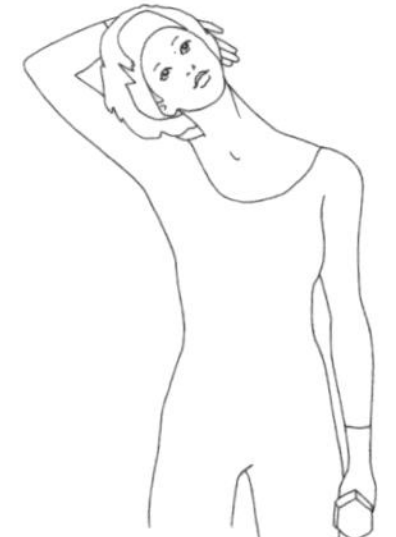

Lateral neck stretch
STRETCH #67

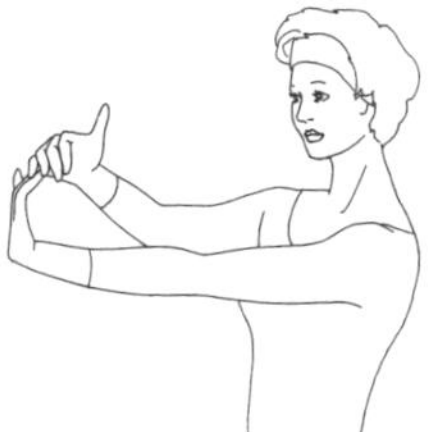

Wrist flexor stretch
STRETCH #69

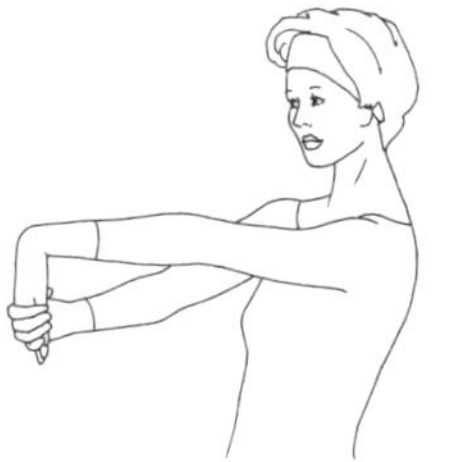

Wrist extensor stretch
STRETCH #70

MARTIAL ARTS

Since "martial arts" describes everything from serene "shadow dancing" to full-contact boxing, it doesn't make sense to give one stretching routine for all forms. The softer styles of martial arts, such as tai chi and Chi Kung, often contain stretches of their own. The following stretch routine is appropriate for more rigorous forms such as karate, kung fu, judo, jujitsu, Thai boxing, and aikido.

Martial arts demands better than average flexibility, strength, and endurance. Many moves also force the muscles to contract at high speeds—in other words, they're ballistic, as the muscles stretch, make contact, and then contract. Since sparring and full-contact fighting contain ballistic motions, some ballistic training makes sense—but not in a warm-up. (Even with warm muscles, it's easy to get injured doing these motions, but the risks increase when muscles are cold.) However, some "old school" martial arts teachers still put quick bouncing and snapping moves into warm-ups. If you find yourself in a class where a teacher warms you up in ways that are painful, you should do your own warm-ups or find another teacher. Warm up your body thoroughly *before* performing any bouncing or snapping motions. Wear all the protective gear you can, and be sure to make stretching an important part of your training routine.

One knee to chest (buttocks, hips, and lower back)

STRETCH #12

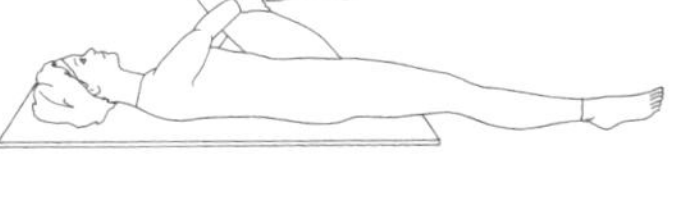

On-your-side quad stretch

STRETCH #19

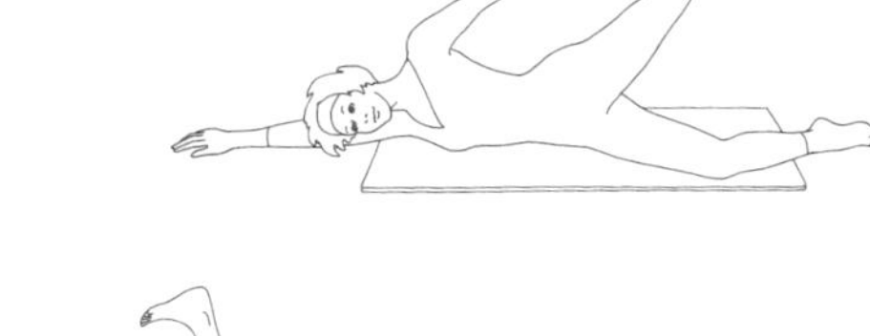

Leg-up hamstring stretch

STRETCH #27

Side-lying groin stretch (inner thigh)

STRETCH #35

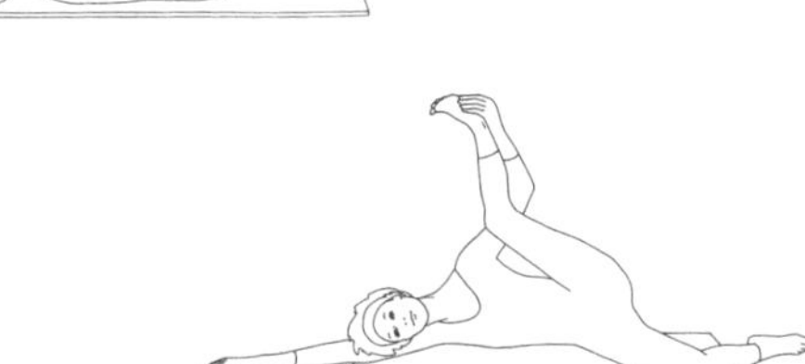

The straddle (inner thigh)
STRETCH #38

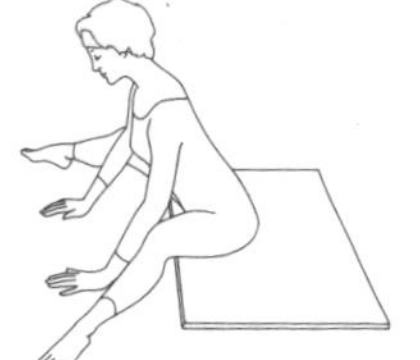

Straddle overhead stretch (obliques and torso)
STRETCH #51

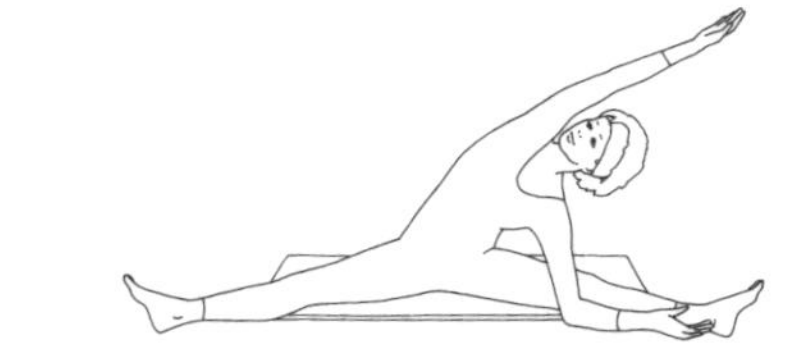

Upward-facing dog (abdominals)
STRETCH #46

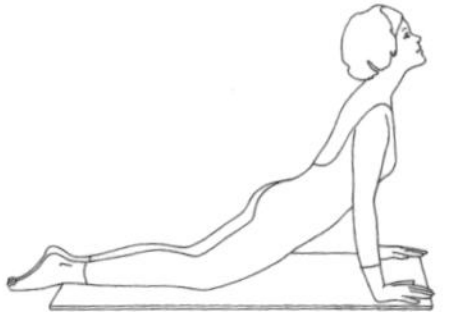

All-fours twist (upper back)
STRETCH #54

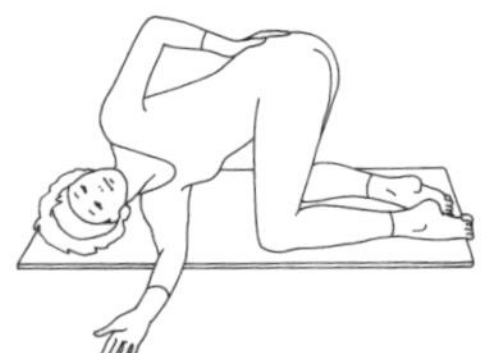

Runner's stretch (hip flexors)
STRETCH #25

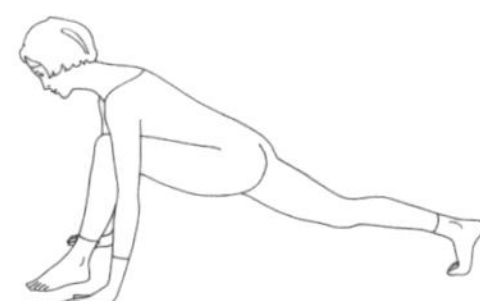

Chest and front-of-shoulder stretch (pole)
STRETCH #81

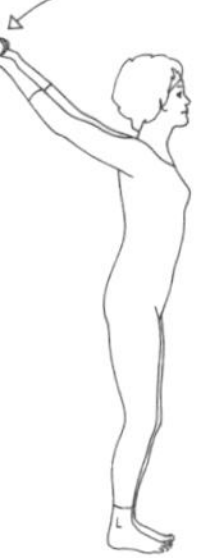

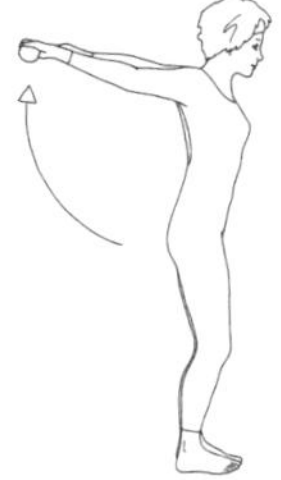

Round-the-world shoulder stretch (pole)

STRETCH #82

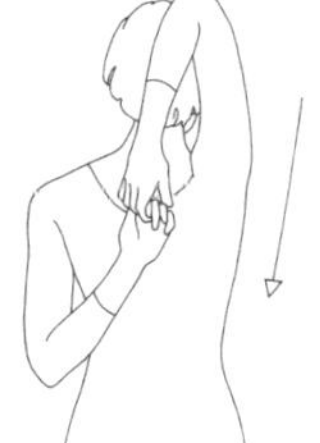

External rotator stretch (shoulders and arms)

STRETCH #62

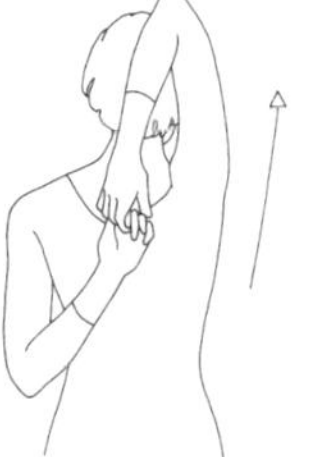

Internal rotator stretch (shoulders and arms)

STRETCH #63

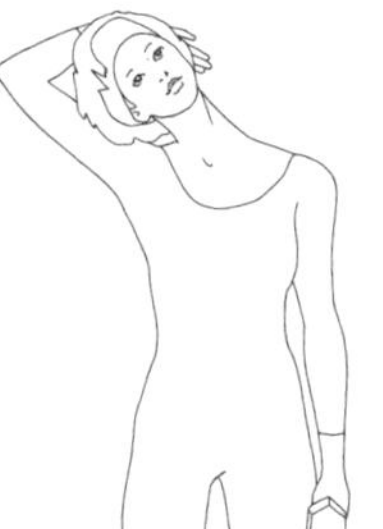

Lateral neck stretch

STRETCH #67

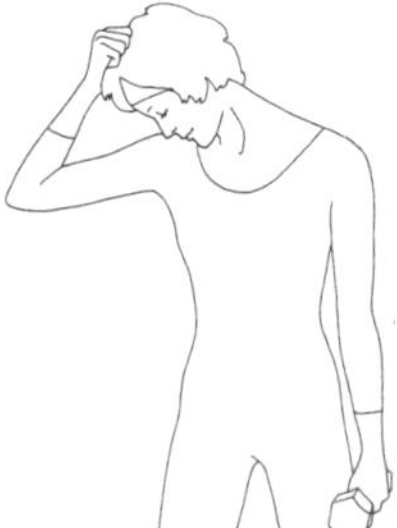

Oblique extensor stretch (neck)

STRETCH #68

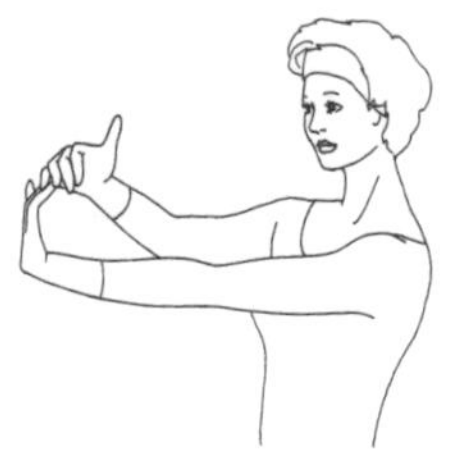

Wrist flexor stretch
STRETCH #69

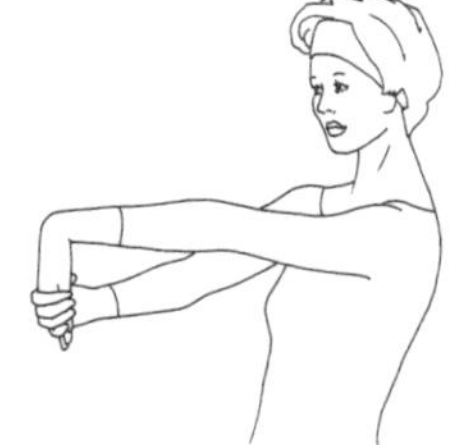

Wrist extensor stretch
STRETCH #70

RACQUET AND BAT SPORTS

Tennis, racquetball, squash, baseball, and softball all use throwing motions for serves and pitches. They also all involve swinging and hitting, which rotate the torso and combine long periods of standing around waiting with quick bursts of motion and sudden directional changes.

To do all of these things well, you need strong arms and flexible shoulders, a flexible lower body to accommodate sudden bursts of energy and changes of direction, plus a stable yet flexible trunk that twists when you hit, pitch, or serve.

Of all the above sports, racquetball and squash are the fastest moving and probably give the best workout—although a rousing game of singles tennis can do the same. But if you're hoping to get fit playing leisurely games of baseball, softball, or doubles tennis, you'd better take a good look at your level of play. If you're not running around for most of the game, you're probably not keeping or getting fit and should supplement these activities with cardiovascular and strength training in addition to stretching.

If you like to stretch before a game, do gentle versions of stretches #1–#12, holding each for just 10 seconds. For a full stretching routine after your game or on days off, do all the stretches but hold each position for 30 seconds.

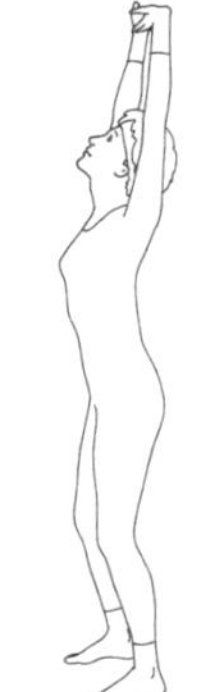

Overhead stretch (obliques and torso)
STRETCH #48

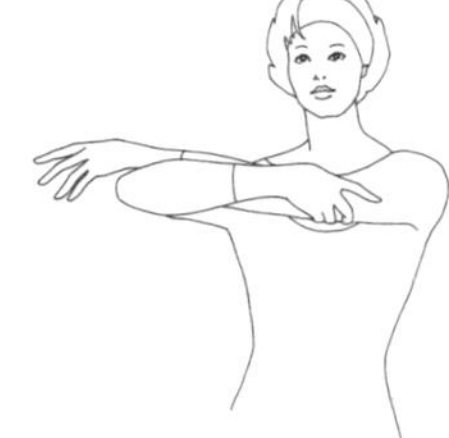

Posterior shoulder stretch
STRETCH #61

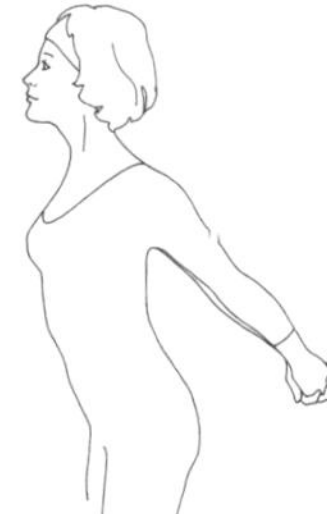

Arms low (chest)
STRETCH #58

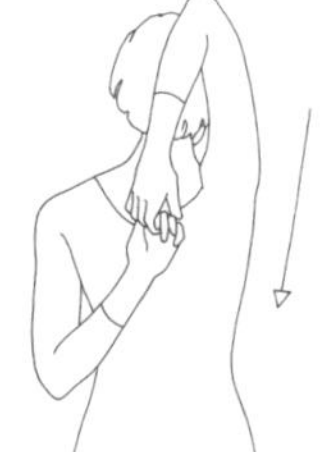

External rotator stretch (shoulders and arms)
STRETCH #62

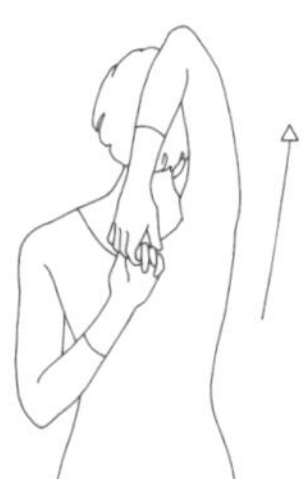

Internal rotator stretch (shoulders and arms)
STRETCH #63

Triceps stretch (shoulders and arms)
STRETCH #64

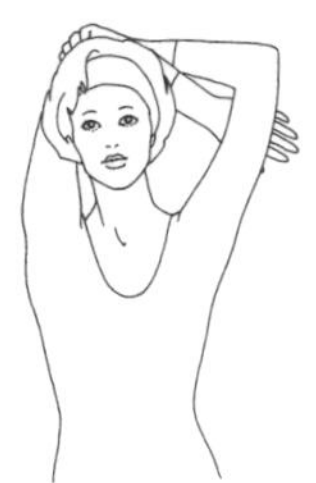

Biceps stretch (shoulders and arms)
STRETCH #65

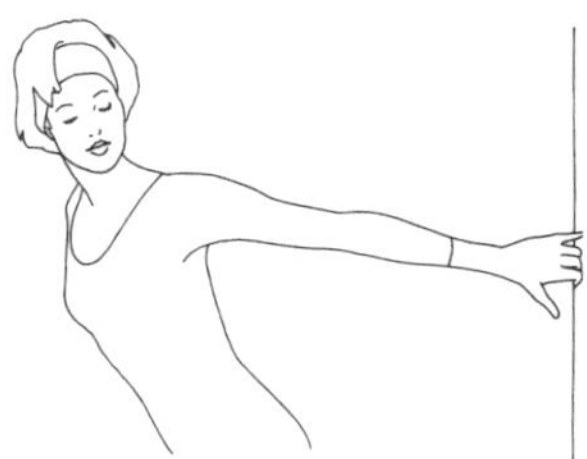

Standing lateral stretch (obliques and torso)
STRETCH #49

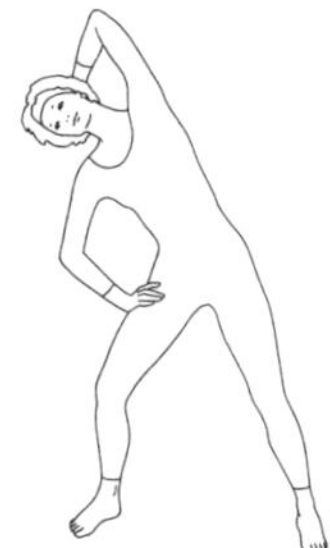

One-arm sit-back stretch (upper back)
STRETCH #56

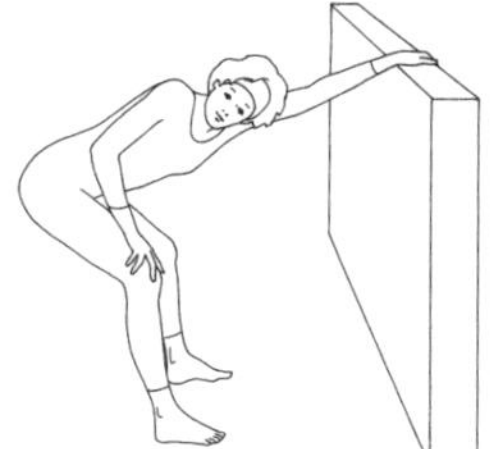

Lateral neck stretch
STRETCH #67

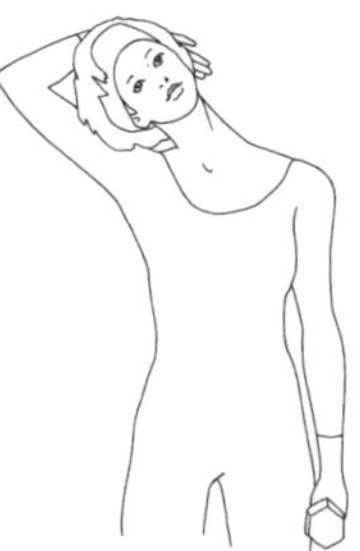

Wrist rotator stretch
STRETCH #71

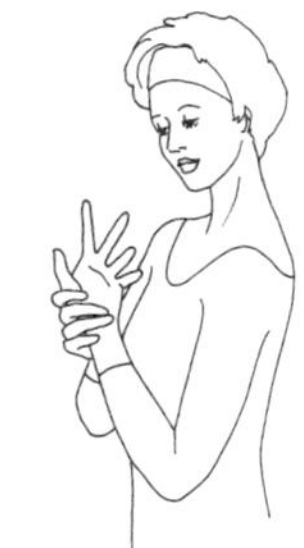

Finger stretches
STRETCH #72

Seated butterfly stretch (inner thigh)
STRETCH #34

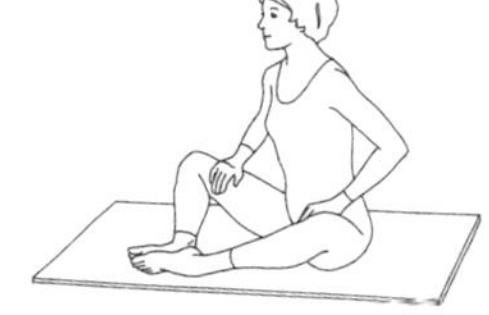

Floor or bench hamstring stretch
STRETCH #29

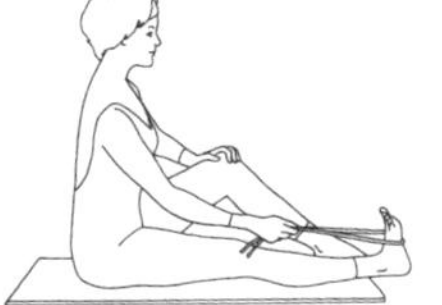

Seated floor twist (buttocks, hips, and lower back)
STRETCH #15

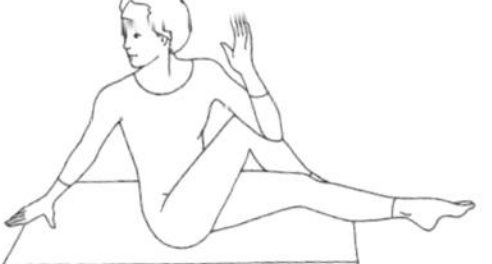

Ankle on the knee (buttocks, hips, and lower back)
STRETCH #14

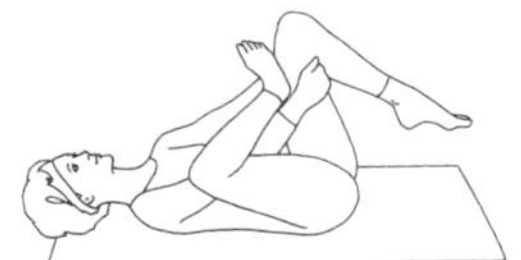

Full-body stretch (abdominals)
STRETCH #45

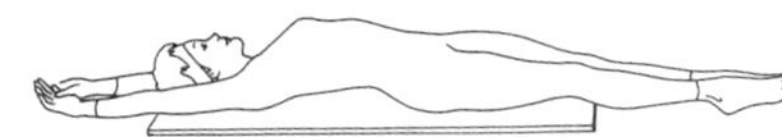

Erector spinae stretch (lower back)
STRETCH #2

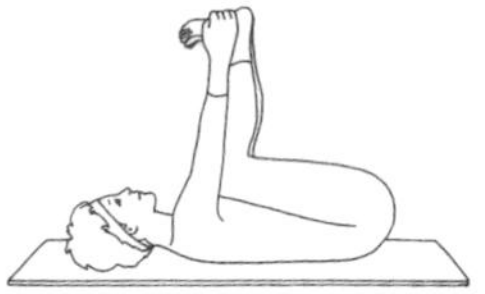

Side-lying floor stretch (outer hip and thigh)
STRETCH #31

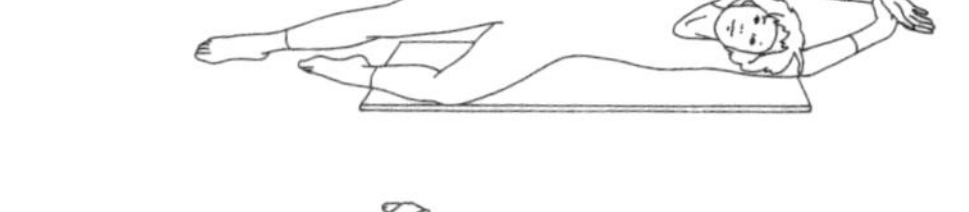

On-your-side quad stretch (quads and hip flexors)
STRETCH #19

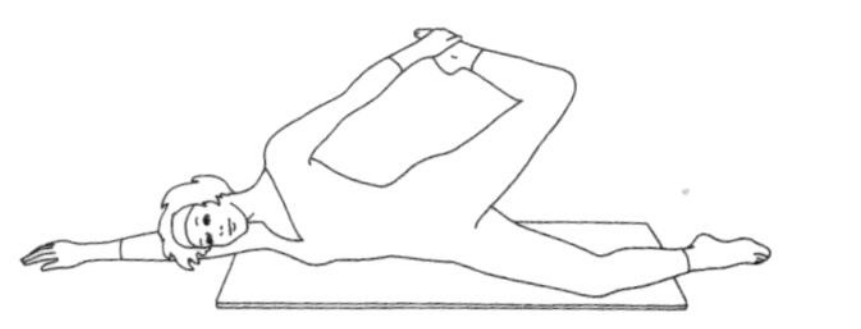

ROWING

Whether you row on a machine or a river, by yourself or with a crew, you're still going to use the same muscles: lats, lower back, upper back, shoulders, chest, arms, abdominals, buttocks, quads, hamstrings, and ankles. Rowing is a beautifully efficient full-body activity that takes (and builds) both endurance and strength. Flexibility is important as well, because many of your motions (especially your forward reach) extend your muscles to their maximum stretching length. To handle this repetitive motion and avoid injury (most common in the lower back and knees), your muscles need to be both flexible and strong.

Erector spinae stretch (lower back)
STRETCH #2

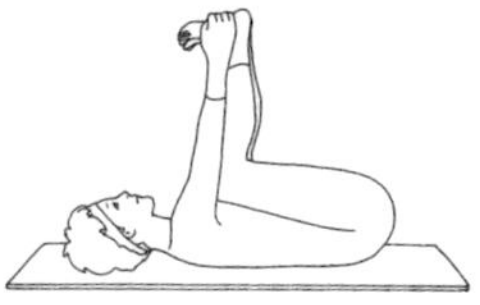

One knee to chest (buttocks, hips, and lower back)
STRETCH #12

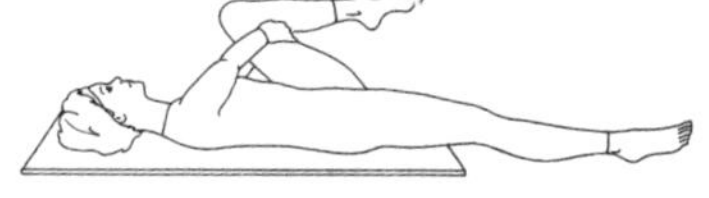

Ankle on the knee (buttocks, hips, and lower back)

STRETCH #14

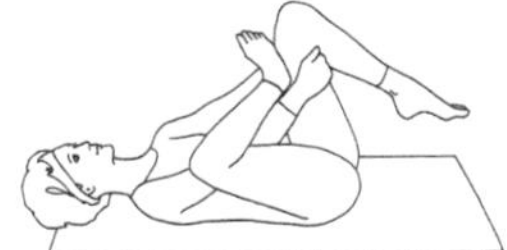

Leg-up hamstring stretch

STRETCH #27

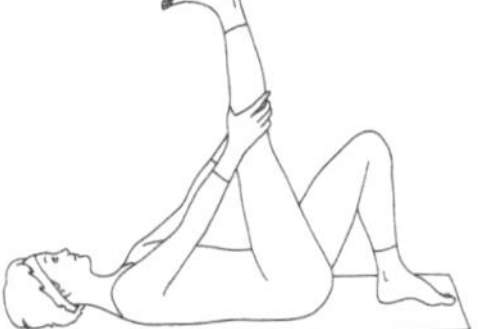

Standing calf stretch

STRETCH #39

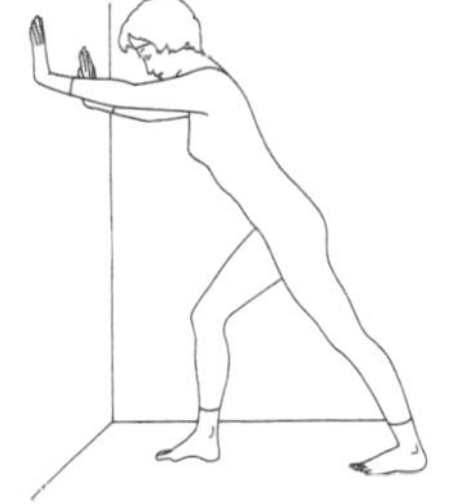

Back-of-the-neck stretch

STRETCH #66

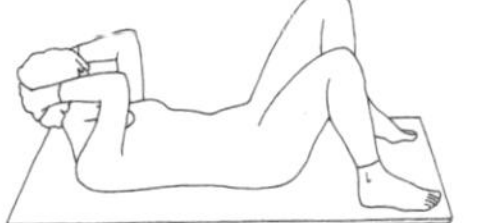

On-your-belly quad stretch

STRETCH #18

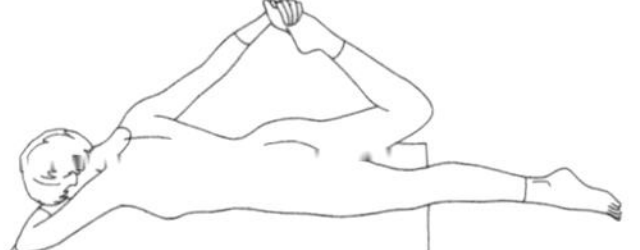

One-half locust (abdominals)

STRETCH #47

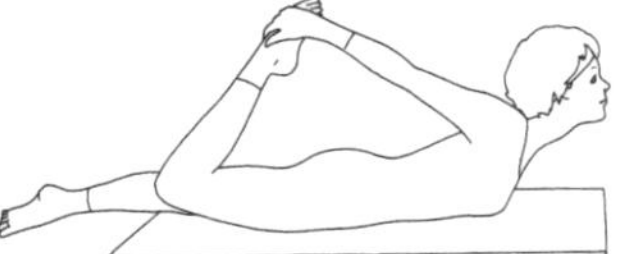

All-fours twist (upper back)

STRETCH #54

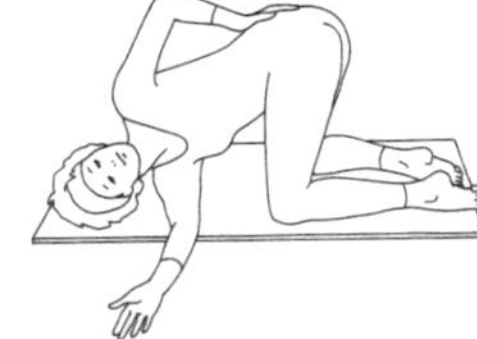

Sit-back stretch (upper back)
STRETCH #55

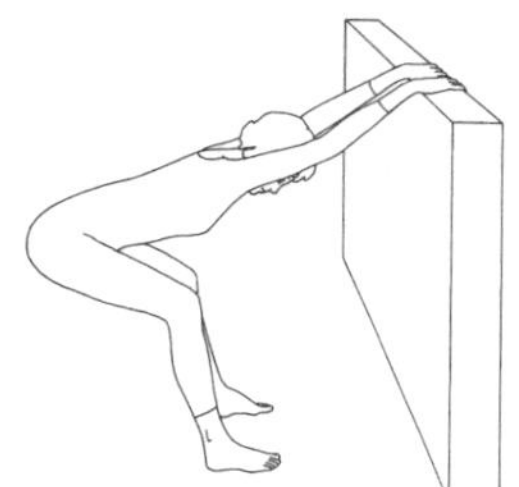

One-arm sit-back stretch (upper back)
STRETCH #56

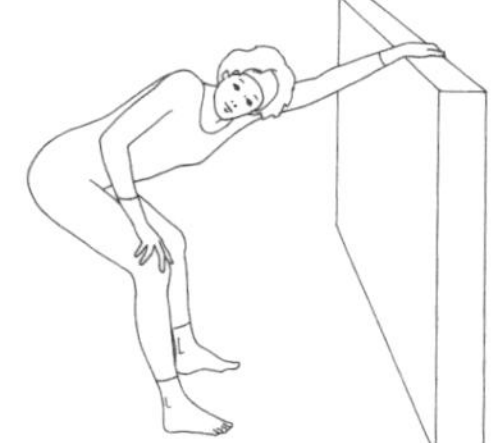

Arms low (chest)
STRETCH #58

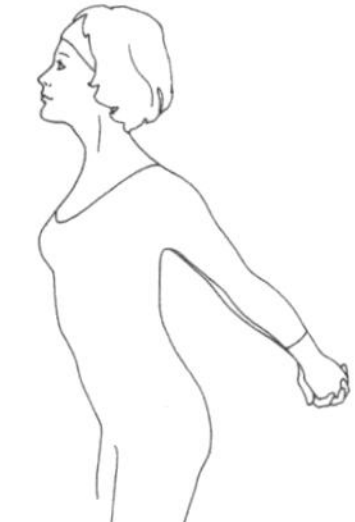

External rotator stretch (shoulders and arms)
STRETCH #62

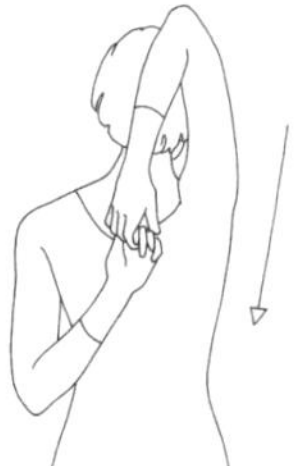

Internal rotator stretch (shoulders and arms)
STRETCH #63

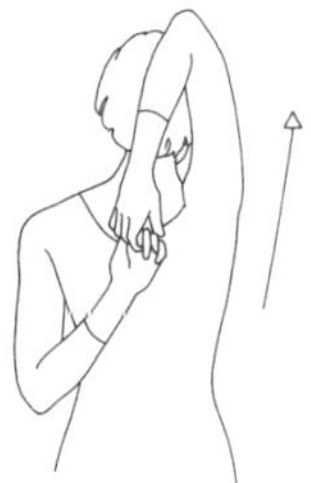

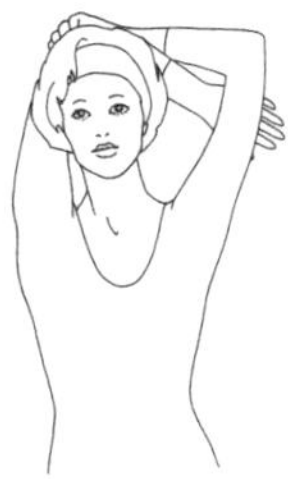

Triceps stretch (shoulders and arms)
STRETCH #64

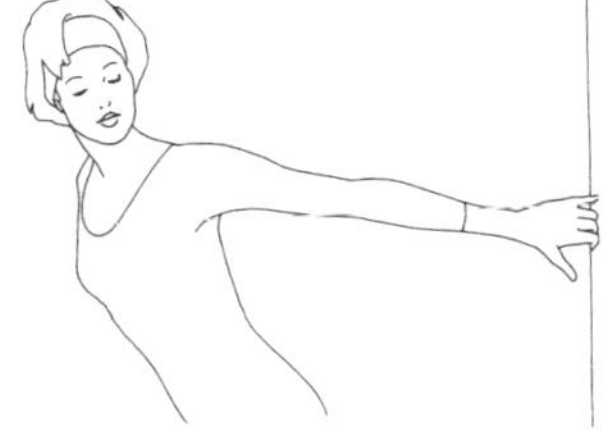

Biceps stretch (shoulders and arms)
STRETCH #65

RUNNING

Whether you race, jog, or shuffle along, stretching can ease the damage running can do to your body. Every time your foot hits the ground, you land with one and a half to five times your body weight, sending shock waves through your entire body. It should come as no surprise then that runners suffer from more overuse injuries than any other athletes. Repetitive pounding also accumulates over time, especially in the ankles, knees, hips, lower back, and shoulders (from pumping the arms). You could run for ten years with no problems and then one day wake up to your body saying "no more." Still, runners tend to be an obsessed group—sometimes running when injured or before an injury fully heals. This, of course, makes matters worse.

If you're committed to running, you should, at the very least, take all the preventative measures you can. Wear good supportive shoes (buy new ones every few months) and run on forgiving surfaces (choose dirt trails over concrete). Undertake strength training for your entire body; don't depend on running for all your leg strength, and add upper-body strength for muscle balance. Be sure to stretch: more flexibility means a longer stride, more efficient use of your muscles, greater speed, a more balanced gait, and more comfort while you run. If you *must* run when injured, do it in the water. (Run in deep water with a buoyant belt and gradually, as you heal, run in progressively more shallow water.)

If you like to stretch before you run, do stretches #1–#8 (hold each for 10 seconds). Be sure to do them again after you run, plus stretches #9–#19 (holding each pose for 10 to 30 seconds).

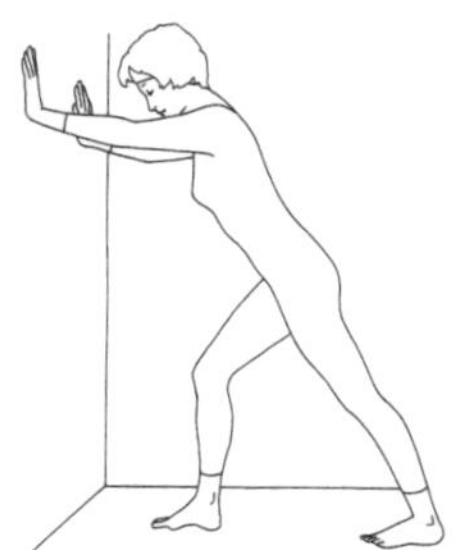

Standing calf stretch
STRETCH #39

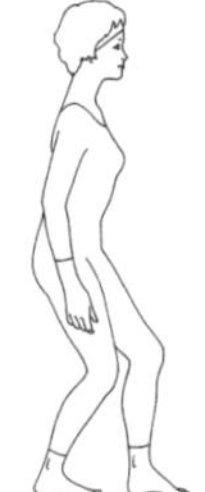

Standing soleus and Achilles stretch
STRETCH #42

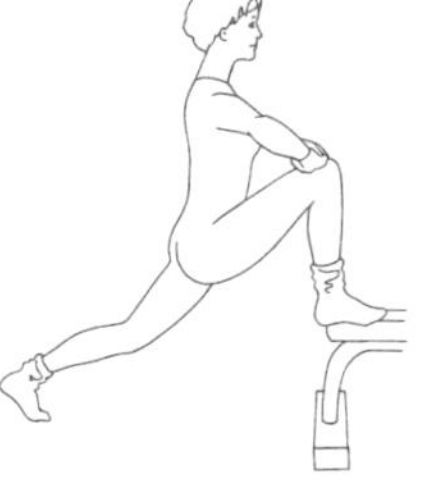

Foot-on-a-step stretch (hip flexors)
STRETCH #26

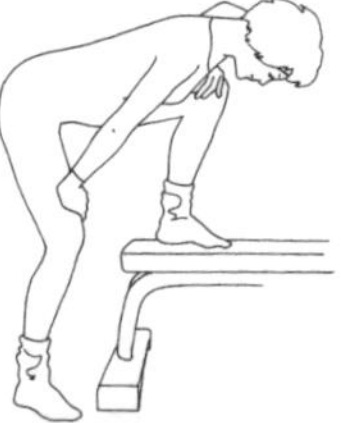

Hang over a chair (inner thigh)
STRETCH #36

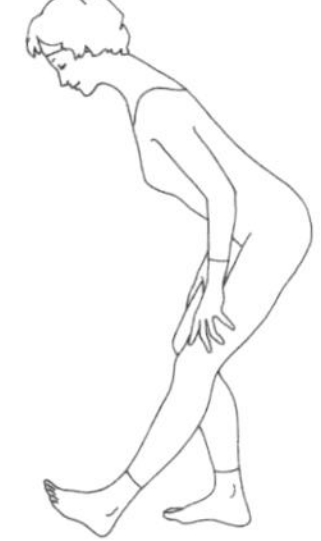

Standing hamstring stretch
STRETCH #30

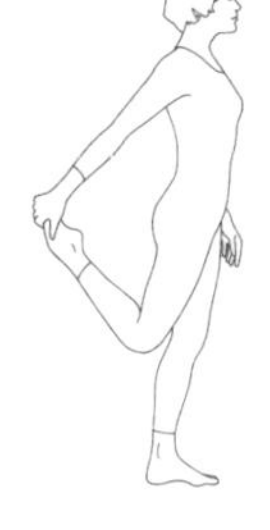

Standing quad stretch
STRETCH #20

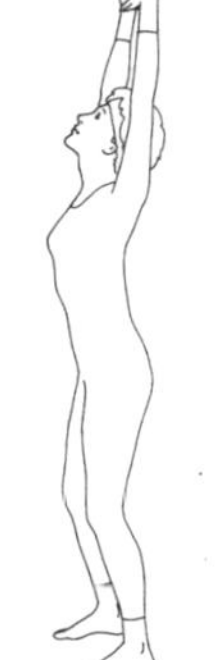

Overhead stretch (shoulders)
STRETCH #48

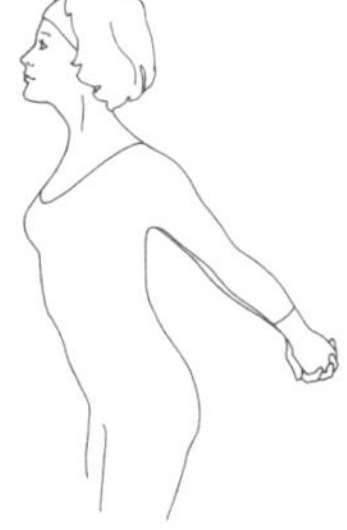

Arms low (chest)
STRETCH #58

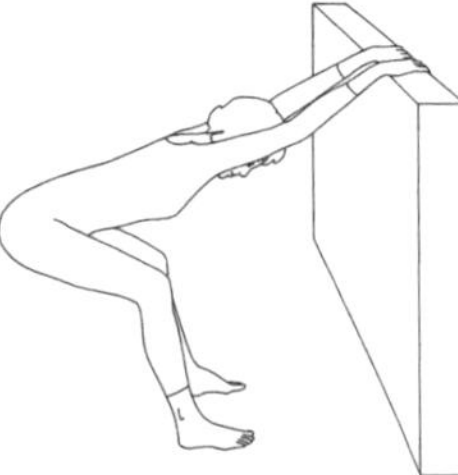

Sit-back stretch (upper back)
STRETCH #55

The full squat (lower back)
STRETCH #11

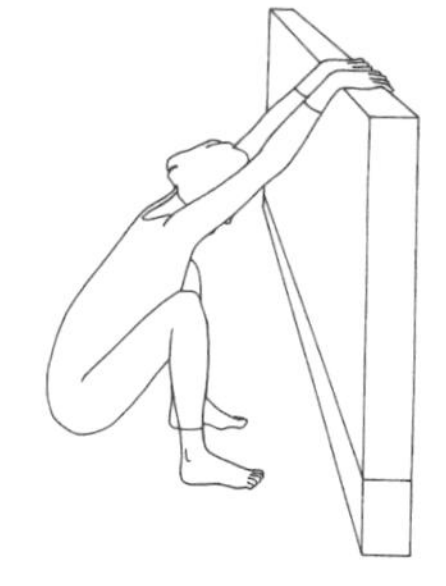

Bench hip flexor stretch
STRETCH #24

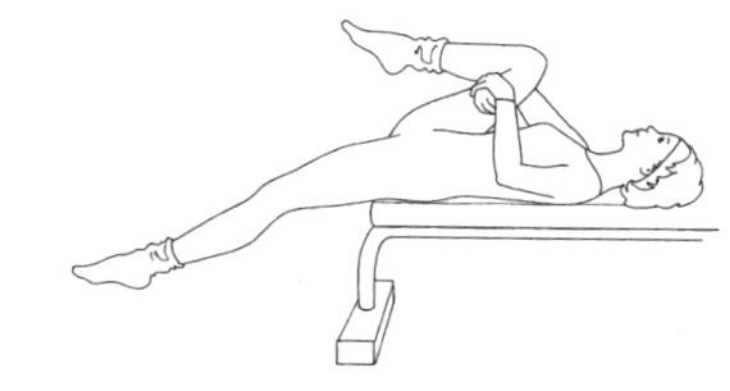

Side-lying stretch on a bench (outer hip and thigh)
STRETCH #32

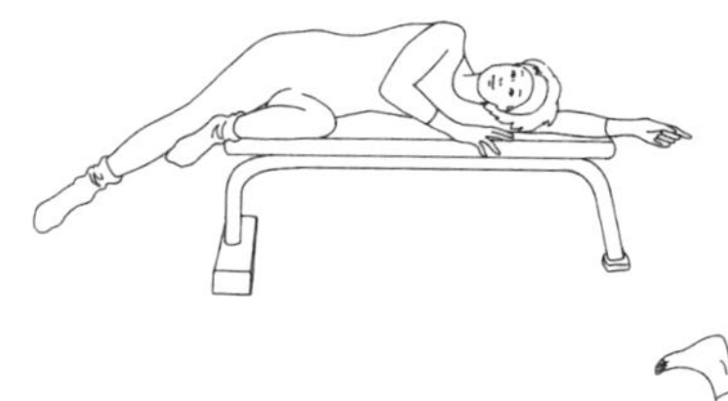

Leg-up hamstring stretch
STRETCH #27

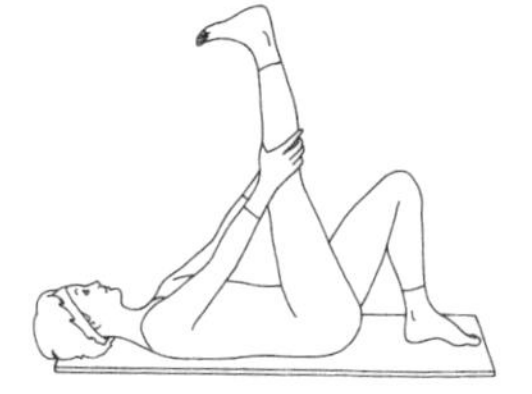

Ankle on the knee (buttocks, hips, and lower back)
STRETCH #14

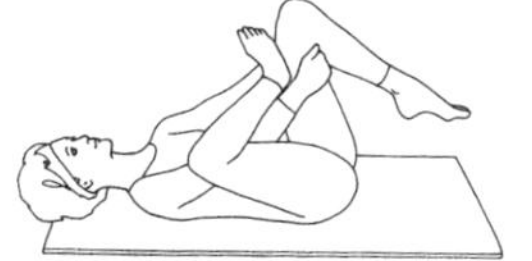

Erector spinae stretch (lower back)
STRETCH #2

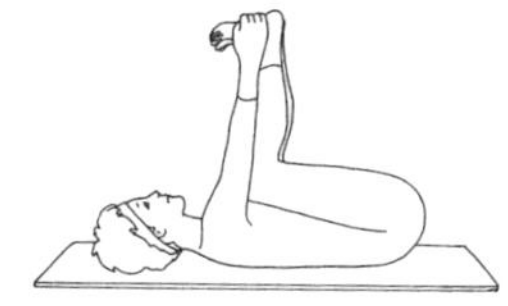

Full-body stretch (abdominals)
STRETCH #45

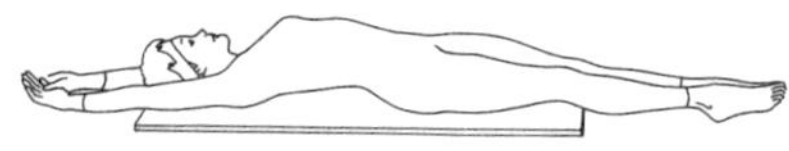

Side-lying groin stretch (inner thigh)
STRETCH #35

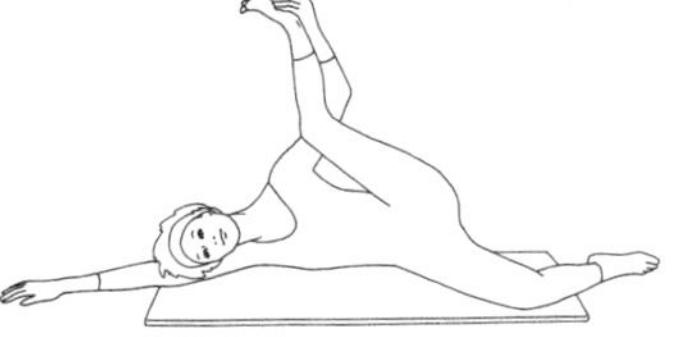

Knee across the body (buttocks, hips, and lower back)
STRETCH #13

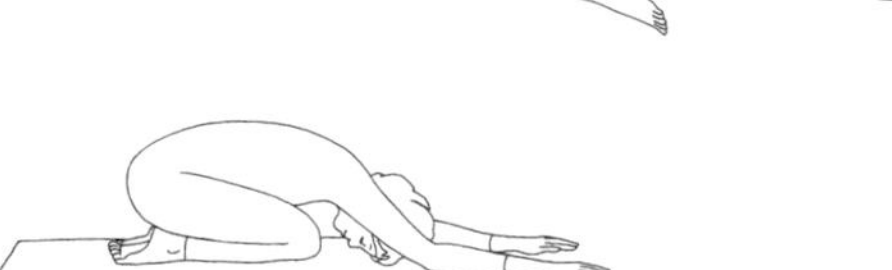

Child's pose (lower back)
STRETCH #6

SKATING

Although professional skaters make it look easy, skating (either on blades or wheels and whether playing hockey, speed skating, or figure skating) takes impressive amounts of coordination, balance, strength, and all-over flexibility. Shifting your weight from leg to leg without falling requires strong and flexible outer and inner thighs, buttocks, quads, hamstrings, and calves. Crouching forward to speed across the ice takes strong abdominals and obliques, flexible hamstrings, and a supple lower back. Jumps, spins, and turns take strong and flexible gluteals, abdominals, inner and outer thighs, torso rotators, neck muscles, shoulders, and arms.

Whatever type of skating you do, skating can be a tremendous workout. It's also a great way to cross-train for ski season. If you skate on wheels, make sure you wear protective pads and a helmet. If you skate on ice, wear elbow pads.

One knee to chest (buttocks, hips, and lower back)
STRETCH #12

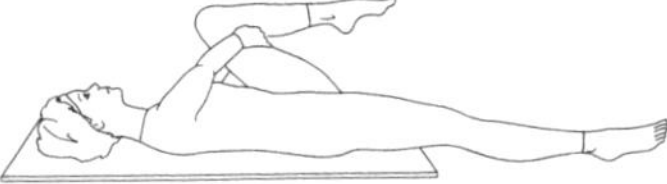

Ankle on the knee (buttocks, hips, and lower back)
STRETCH #14

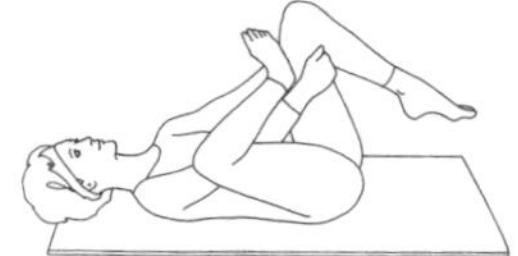

Knee across the body (buttocks, hips, and lower back)
STRETCH #13

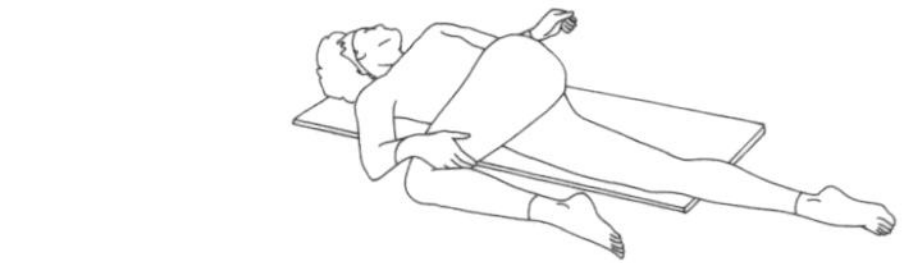

Side-lying floor stretch (outer hip and thigh)
STRETCH #31

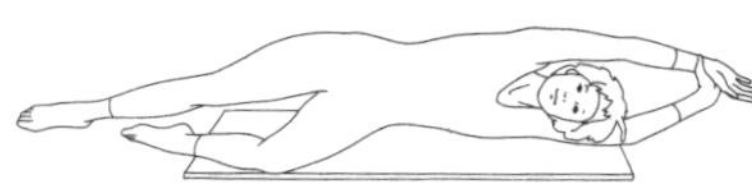

On-your-side quad stretch
STRETCH #19

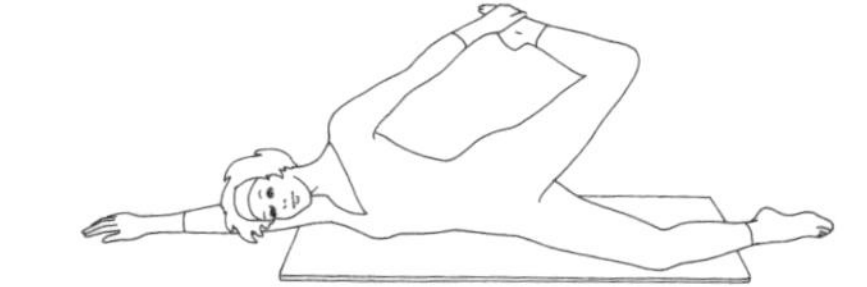

Dancer's stretch (buttocks, hips, and lower back)
STRETCH #16

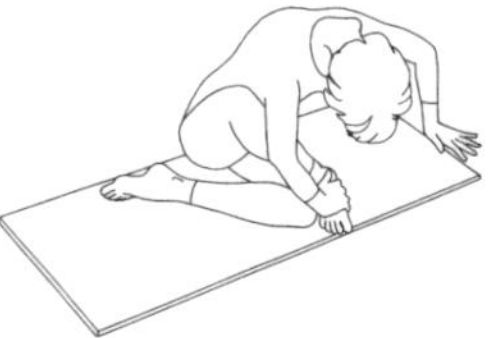

Floor or bench hamstring stretch
STRETCH #29

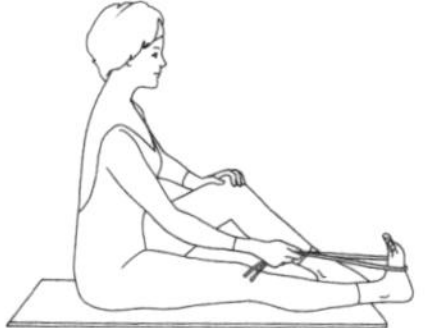

Seated calf stretch
STRETCH #41

The straddle (inner thigh)
STRETCH #38

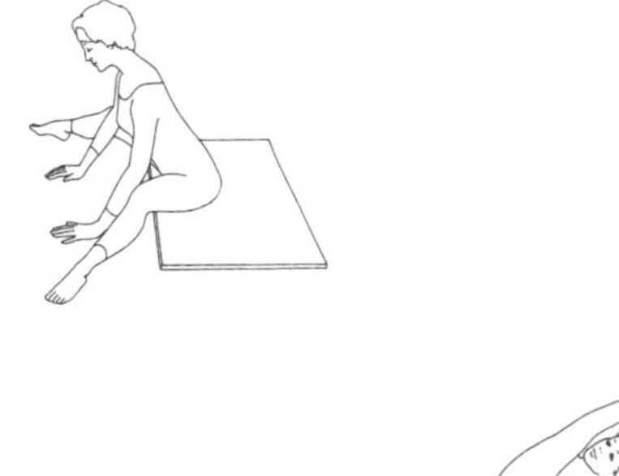

Straddle overhead stretch (obliques and torso)
STRETCH #51

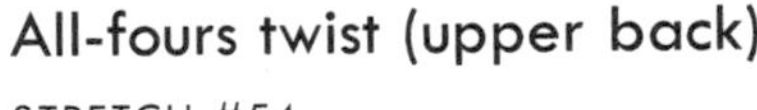

All-fours twist (upper back)
STRETCH #54

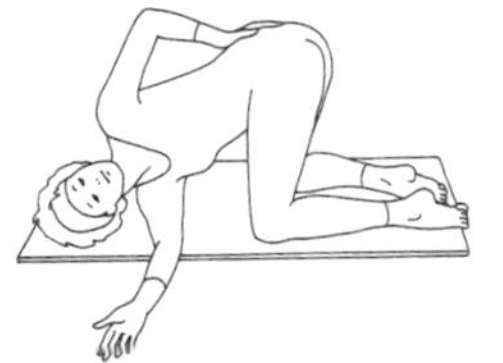

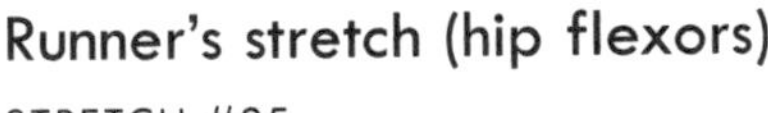

Runner's stretch (hip flexors)
STRETCH #25

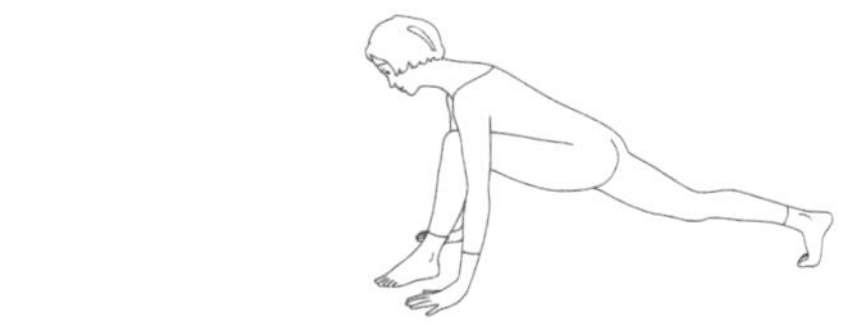

Child's pose (lower back)
STRETCH #6

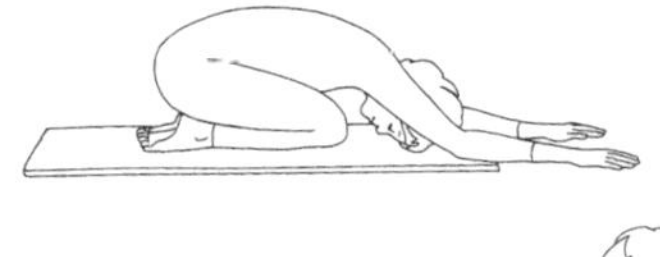

Arms low (chest)
STRETCH #58

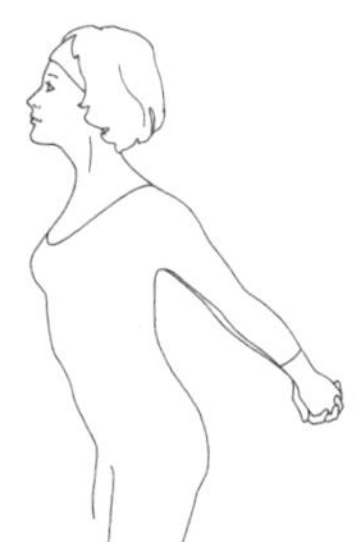

Posterior shoulder stretch
STRETCH #61

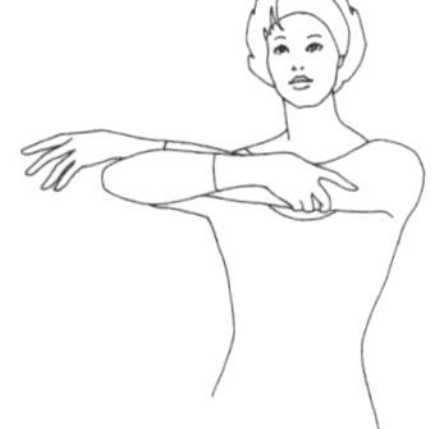

Lateral neck stretch
STRETCH #67

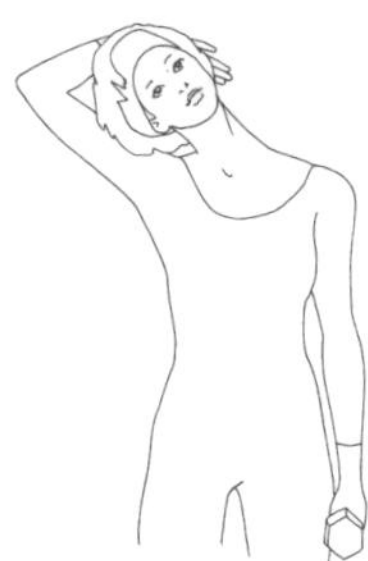

SKIING AND SNOWBOARDING

To be a decent skier (downhill and cross-country) or snowboarder, you need agility—a combination of strength, endurance, and flexibility. These sports all combine "push-off" (strength) moves, which use the hamstrings, gluteals, and quads with "floating" motions in which the knees, hips, and torso absorb the shock of bouncing over the snow. You use your bigger muscles to propel yourself forward and your smaller muscles to maintain your balance, shift your weight, turn, and stop. The more conditioned and flexible you are in muscles both big and small, the more efficient these motions become. The end result is that you can have more fun and look more graceful, too.

Although you might think skiing and snowboarding are lower-body sports, they also use the torso, shoulders, and arms. But if you want a workout while you play in the snow, you should know that even though downhill skiing and snowboarding can build leg strength and muscular endurance, they do *not* build cardiovascular endurance. Cross-country skiing, however, is still one of the best aerobic workouts around. To be all-over fit, supplement the sport of your choice with activities that provide what it cannot.

If you like to warm up and stretch before you hit the slopes, do stretches #1–#12 before your first run of the day. Do stretches #13–#23 after skiing, preferably in front of a fire. Stretching after you ski is especially important if you exercise only during ski season, since unused muscles get sore sooner and stay sore longer. Stretching can minimize your postskiing pain.

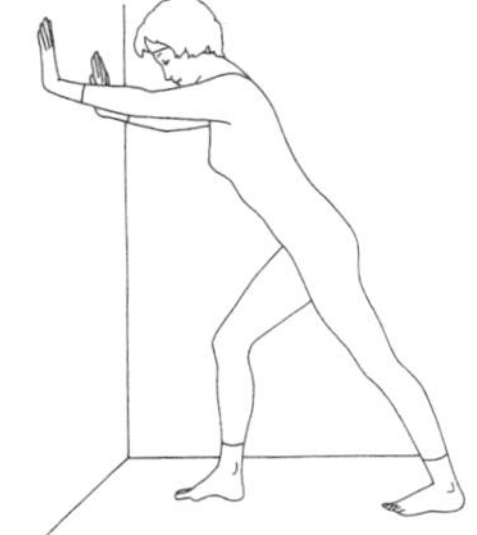

Standing calf stretch
STRETCH #39

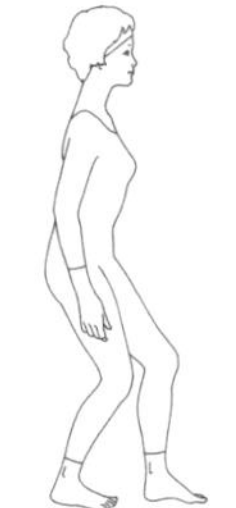

Standing soleus and Achilles stretch
STRETCH #42

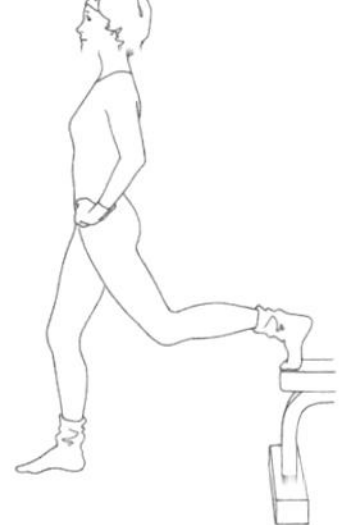

Standing elevated quad stretch (quads and hip flexors)
STRETCH #22

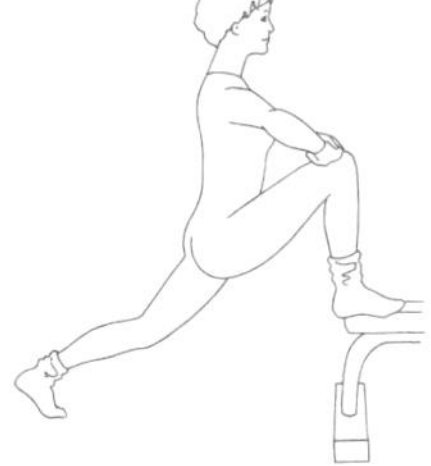

Foot-on-a-step stretch (hip flexors)
STRETCH #26

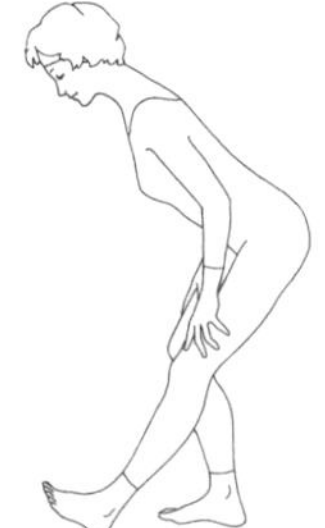

Standing hamstring stretch
STRETCH #30

Standing pelvic tilt (lower back)
STRETCH #8

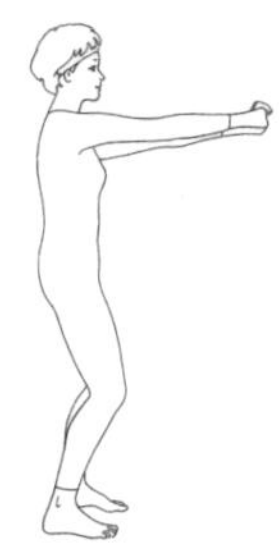

Sit-back stretch (upper back)
STRETCH #55

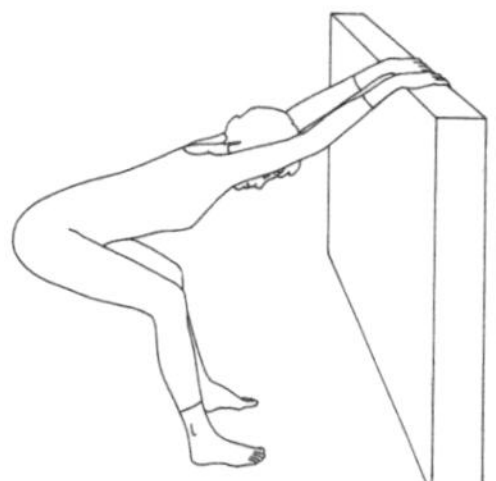

Overhead stretch (obliques and torso)
STRETCH #48

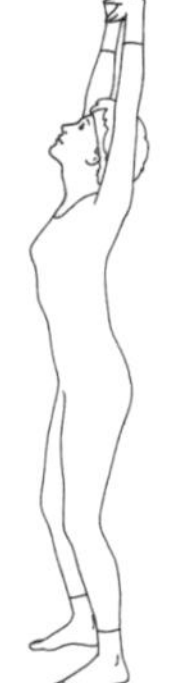

Standing lateral stretch (obliques and torso)
STRETCH #49

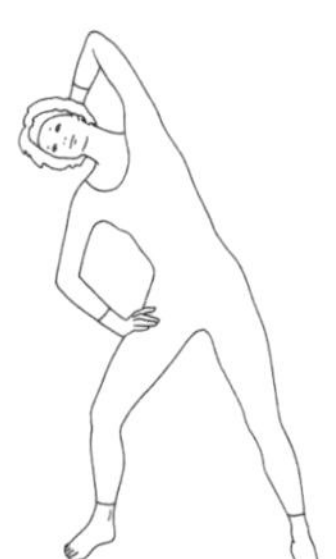

Arms low (chest)
STRETCH #58

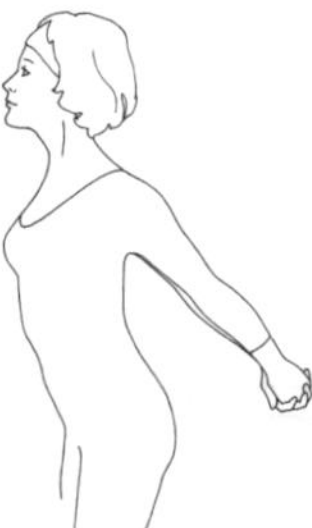

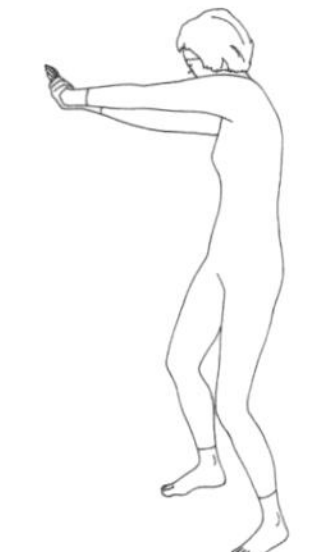

Side wrist pull (upper back)
STRETCH #53

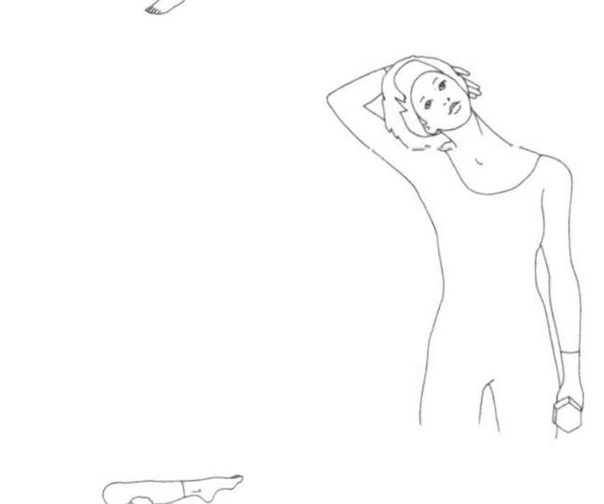

Lateral neck stretch
STRETCH #67

One knee to chest (buttocks, hips, and lower back)
STRETCH #12

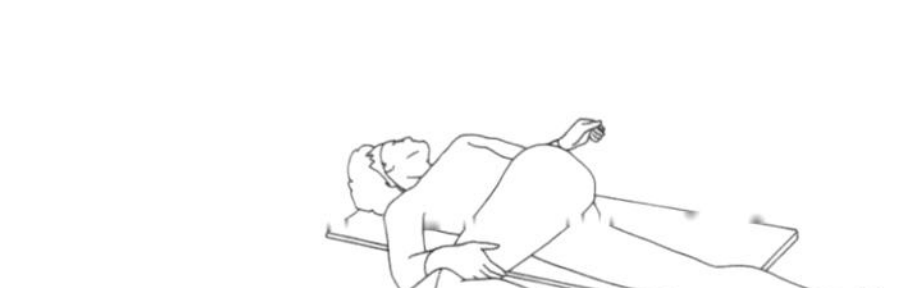

Knee across the body (buttocks, hips, and lower back)
STRETCH #13

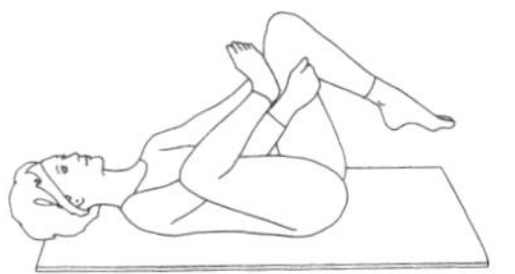

Ankle on the knee (buttocks, hips, and lower back)
STRETCH #14

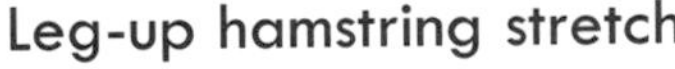

Leg-up hamstring stretch
STRETCH #27

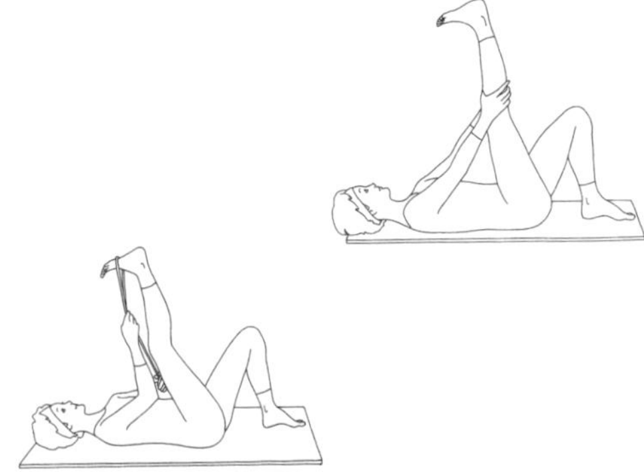

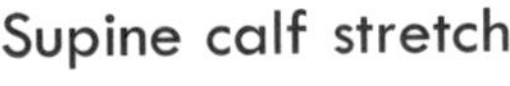

Supine calf stretch
STRETCH #40

Full-body stretch (abdominals)
STRETCH #45

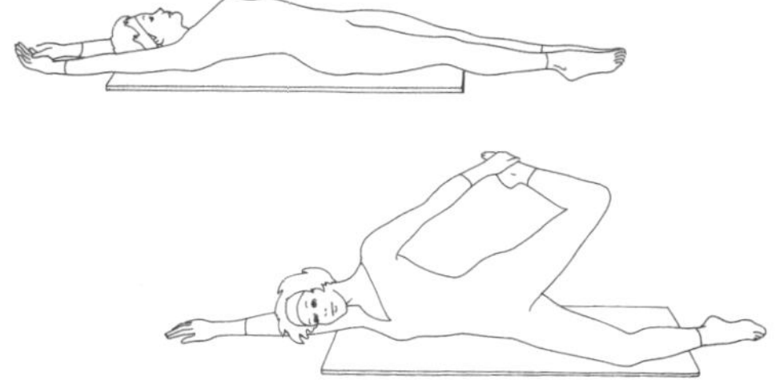

On-your-side quad stretch
STRETCH #19

Side-lying floor stretch (outer hip and thigh)
STRETCH #31

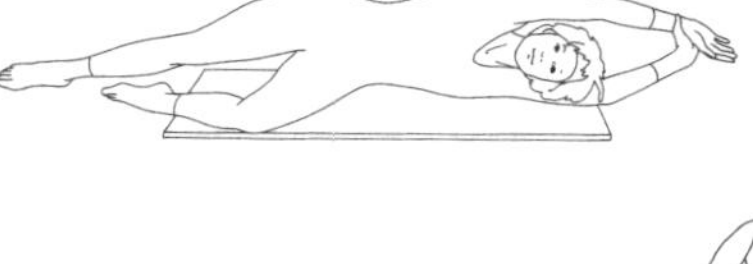

Seated overhead stretch (obliques and torso)
STRETCH #50

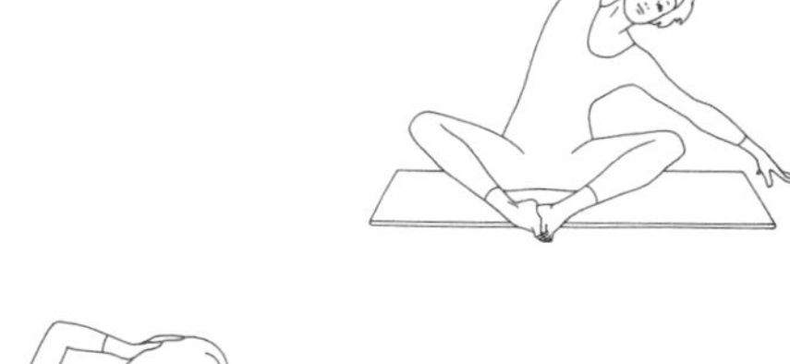

All-fours twist (upper back)
STRETCH #54

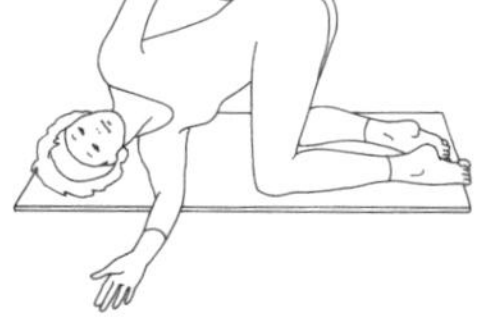

Child's pose (lower back)
STRETCH #6

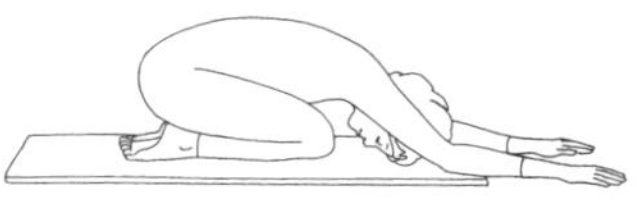

SOCCER

If you're not in shape before you hit the soccer field, you'll wish you were. Soccer is a highly demanding sport; you don't simply need strength, endurance, and flexibility—you need them in the extreme. You need the speed of a sprinter, the endurance of a marathoner, the explosive acceleration of a football running back, the ability to quickly change directions of a tennis player, the leaping skills of a volleyball player, and the accurate and powerful kicks of a black belt in tae kwon do.

Unfortunately, having to perform these different motions also puts soccer players at high risk for injuries. Groins, hamstrings, knees, and calves are especially vulnerable. So are necks and heads—and collisions are part of the game. To preserve your life as a player, stay in shape, warm up, stretch lightly before you play, and stretch deeply after the game and on days off to minimize postgame soreness.

More advanced standing pelvic tilt (lower back)
STRETCH #9

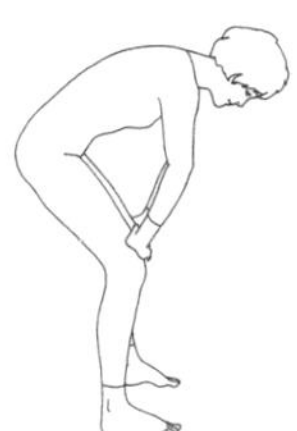

Standing quad stretch
STRETCH #20

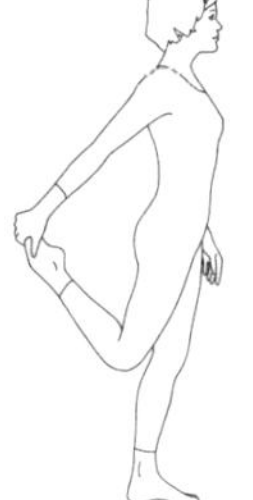

Foot-on-a-step stretch (hip flexors)
STRETCH #26

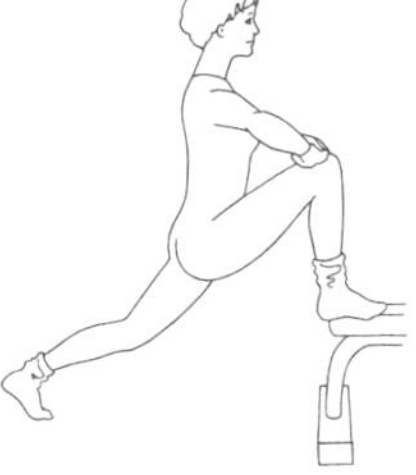

Standing hamstring stretch
STRETCH #30

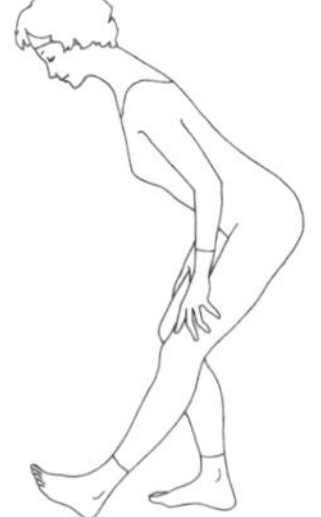

Standing inner-thigh stretch

STRETCH #37

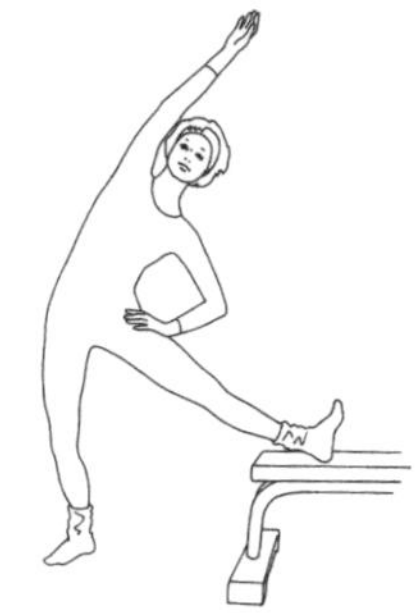

Standing side hip stretch (outer hip and thigh)

STRETCH #33

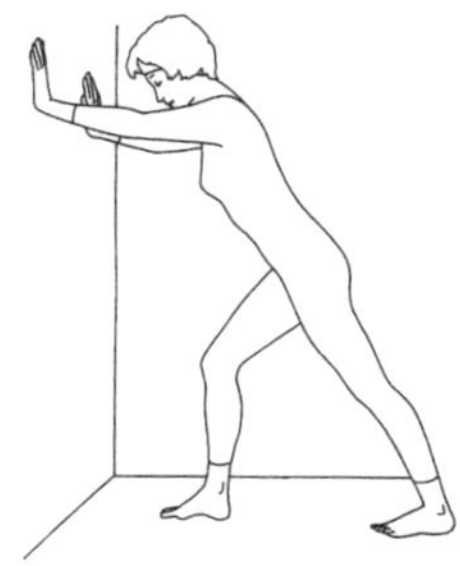

Standing calf stretch

STRETCH #39

Standing soleus and Achilles stretch

STRETCH #42

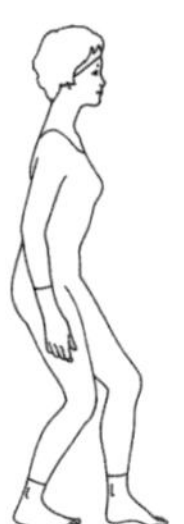

Overhead stretch (obliques and torso)

STRETCH #48

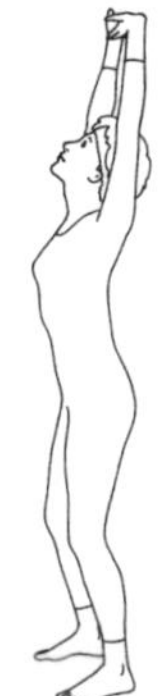

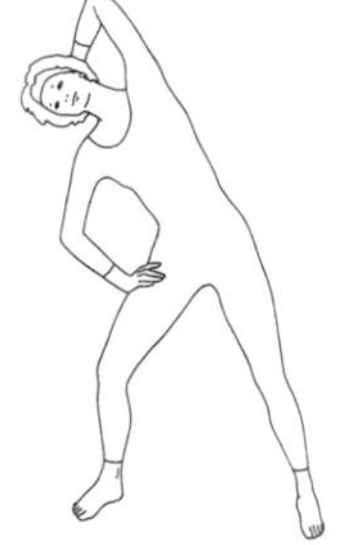

Standing lateral stretch (obliques and torso)
STRETCH #49

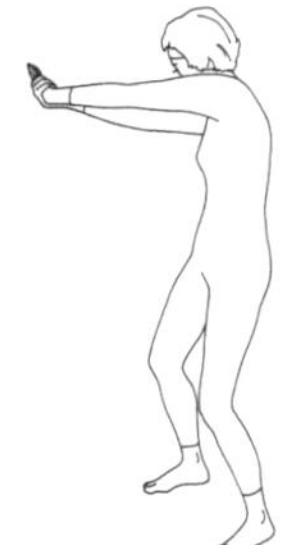

Side wrist pull (upper back)
STRETCH #53

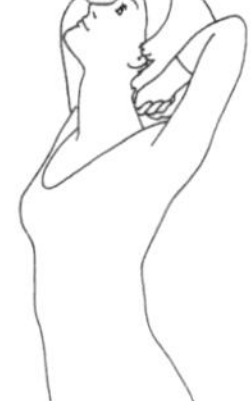

Hands behind your head (chest and front of shoulders)
STRETCH #57

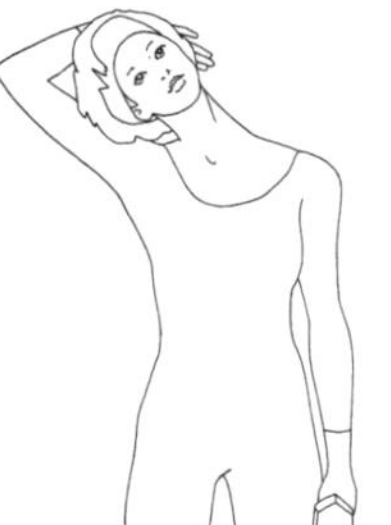

Lateral neck stretch
STRETCH #67

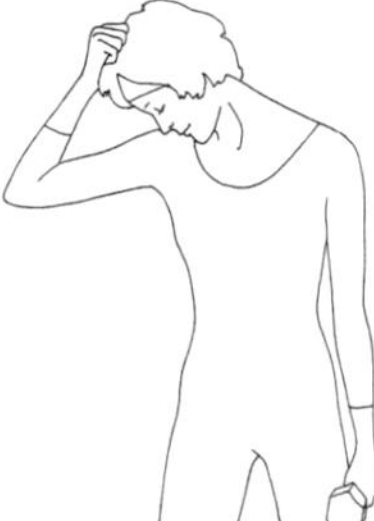

Oblique extensor stretch (neck)
STRETCH #68

Back-of-the-neck stretch
STRETCH #66

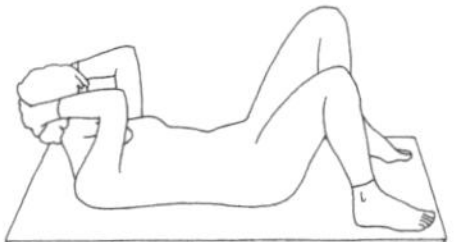

Flex and point (ankles and feet)
STRETCH #73

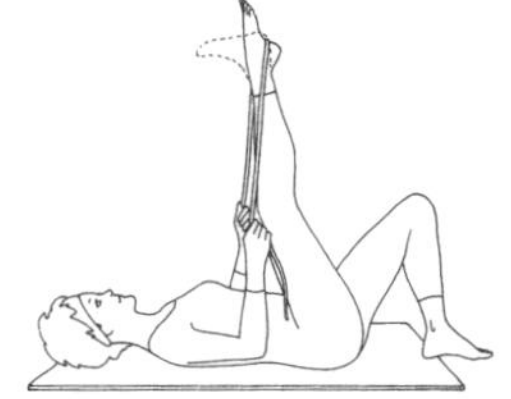

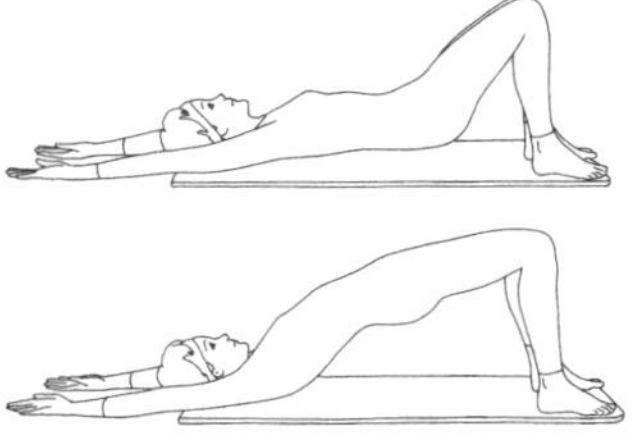

Pelvic tilt into bridge (lower back)
STRETCH #7

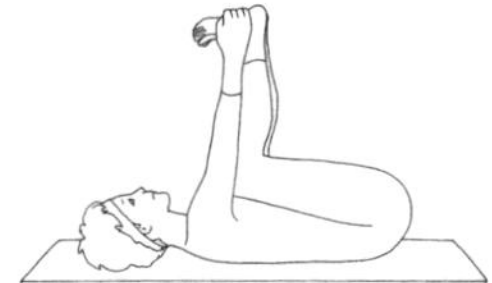

Erector spinae stretch (lower back)
STRETCH #2

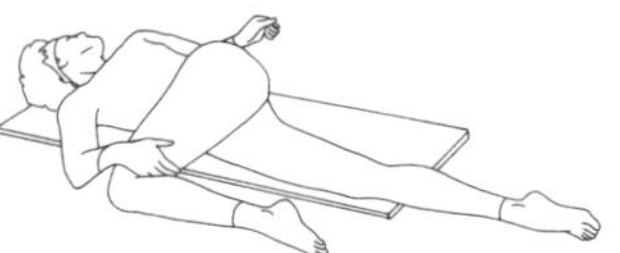

Knee across the body (buttocks, hips, and lower back)
STRETCH #13

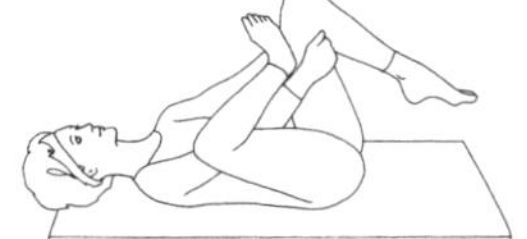

Ankle on the knee (buttocks, hips, and lower back)
STRETCH #14

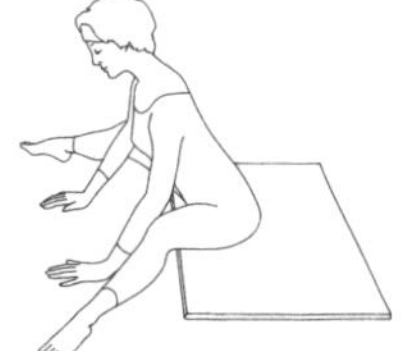

The straddle (inner thigh)
STRETCH #38

Straddle overhead stretch (obliques and torso)
STRETCH #51

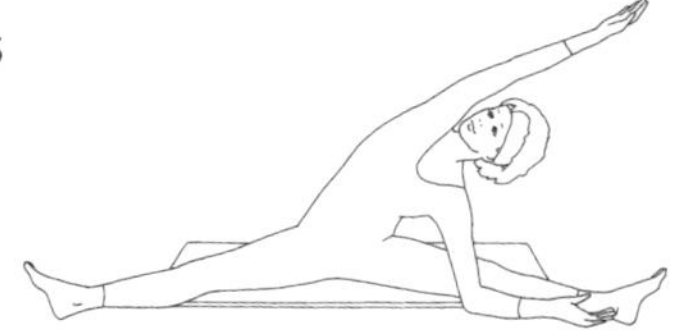

SWIMMING

Moving your near-weightless body through water (which has twelve times the resistance of air) both strengthens and stretches your muscles at the same time. In the water, almost everyone is more flexible, since muscles don't have to fight gravity. But to carry that flexibility onto dry land, you need to stretch on land as well.

Swimmers mostly need a healthy range of motion in the shoulder joint (a problematic area—many people have limitations here). Over time, however, even an injured shoulder can regain its previous flexibility with a good stretching program. Better shoulder flexibility leads to a more efficient stroke, less wear and tear on the joint, and greater swimming speed.

Swimming is not just an upper-body sport. A strong, stable, and flexible torso can help you roll from side to side and cut through the water efficiently when you swim. Flopping back and forth in the water slows you down and wastes energy. Strong, flexible ankles, knees, and hips give you a powerful kick. A flexible neck allows you to turn and breathe when you do the crawl.

Although swimming is good for your heart and muscles, it's not the best way to strengthen your skeleton. If swimming is your only form of exercise, you should add some activity where gravity is more at play as well to increase your bone density. Walking and weight lifting can help swimmers strengthen bones.

If you like to stretch before you swim, do stretches #1–#12, holding each for 10 seconds. These stretches work best, however, when your muscles are warm *after* you exercise.

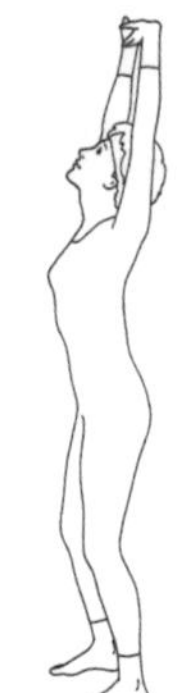

Overhead stretch (obliques and torso)
STRETCH #48

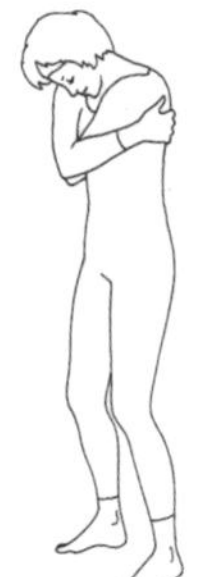

Hug yourself (upper back)
STRETCH #52

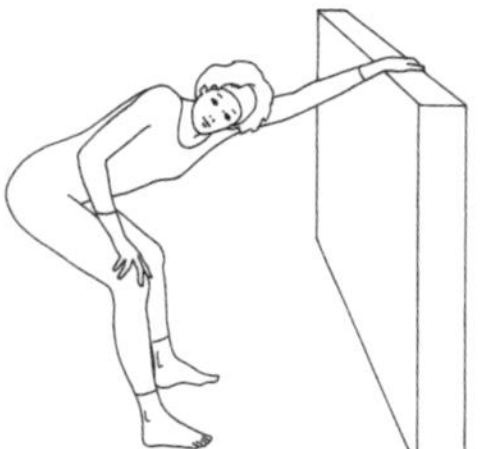

One-arm sit-back stretch (upper back)
STRETCH #56

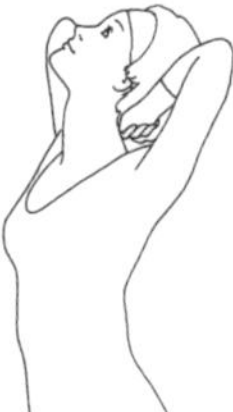

Hands behind your head (chest and front of shoulders)
STRETCH #57

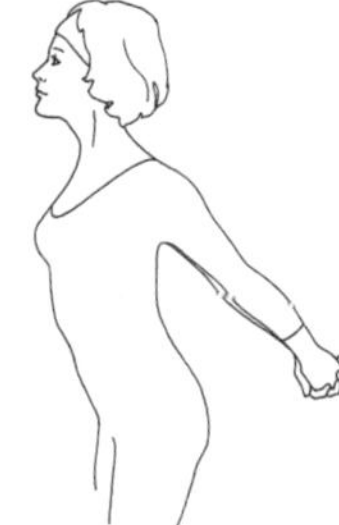

Arms low (chest)
STRETCH #58

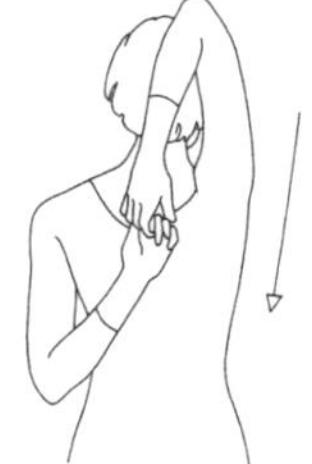

External rotator stretch (shoulders and arms)
STRETCH #62

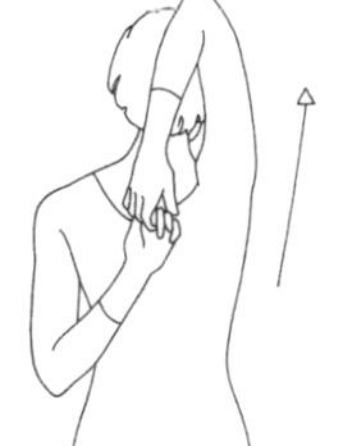

Internal rotator stretch (shoulders and arms)
STRETCH #63

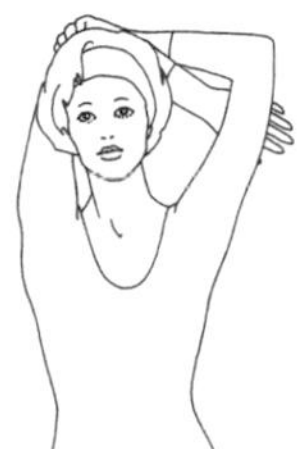

Triceps stretch (shoulders and arms)
STRETCH #64

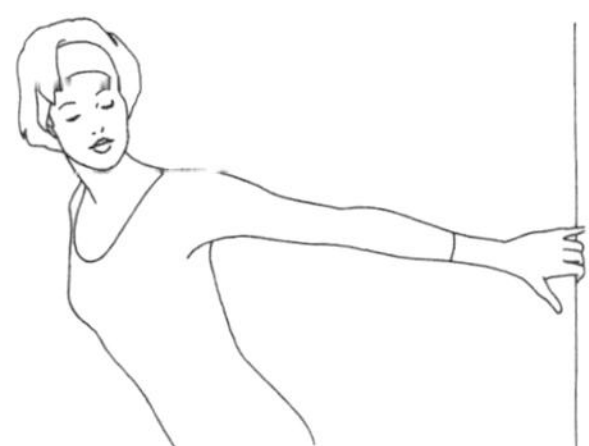

Biceps stretch (shoulders and arms)
STRETCH #65

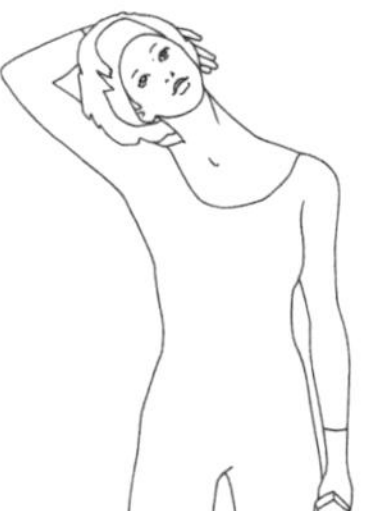

Lateral neck stretch
STRETCH #67

Wrist flexor stretch

STRETCH #69

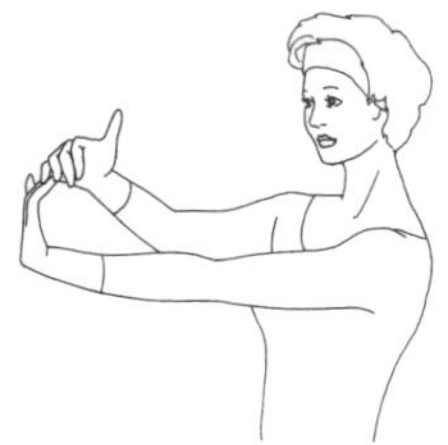

Erector spinae stretch (lower back)

STRETCH #2

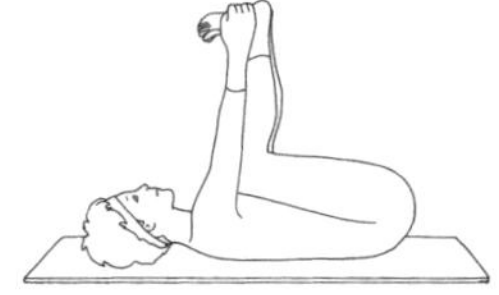

Full-body stretch (abdominals)

STRETCH #45

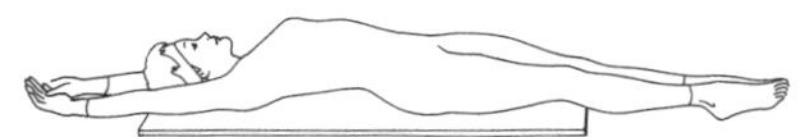

Leg-up hamstring stretch

STRETCH #27

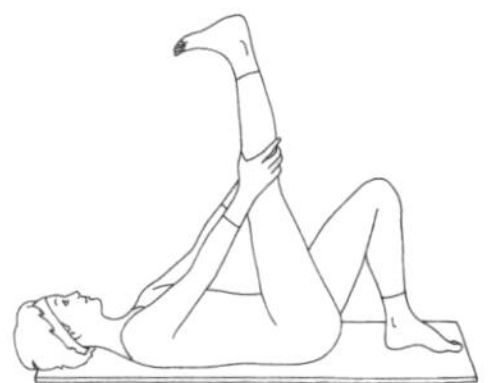

Flex and point (ankles and feet)

STRETCH #73

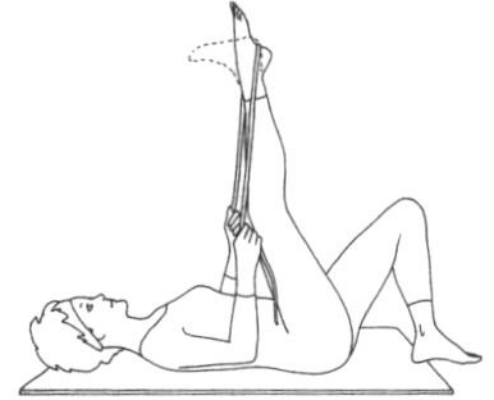

Inner-ankle stretch

STRETCH #75

Outer-ankle stretch

STRETCH #76

Side-lying floor stretch (outer hip and thigh)
STRETCH #31

On-your-side quad stretch (quads and hip flexors)
STRETCH #19

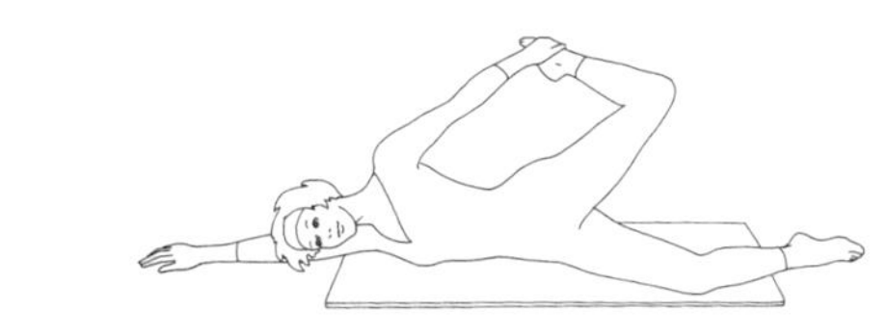

Seated butterfly stretch (inner thigh)
STRETCH #34

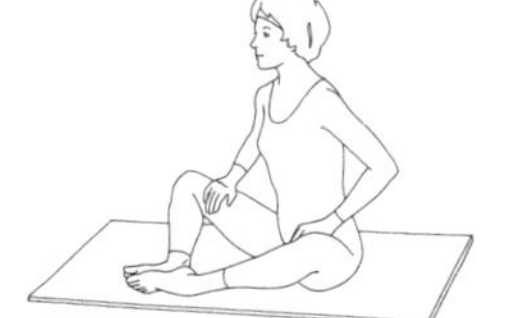

VOLLEYBALL

Muhammad Ali could have been talking about volleyball when he said, "Float like a butterfly, sting like bee." Whether you play on a court or in the sand or dirt, volleyball is a great sport and a challenging workout. One moment, you can feel like a dancer; the next, all your killer instincts come out. To play well, you have to push your body to its limits, leap, twist, spike, lean forward and back, and occasionally fall on your knees or butt. Being flexible allows you to change from butterfly into bee and back again without broadcasting your moves too soon or hurting yourself in the process.

Since volleyball is so strenuous, it can take a toll on the hips, knees, and ankles—and also on the shoulders, arms, and wrists. Maintaining flexibility in these areas can both prevent injuries and improve your game.

If you like to stretch before a match, do stretches #1–#14, but hold each for only 10 seconds. Do them again, plus stretches #15–#19, after your games and on days off, holding each one for 30 seconds.

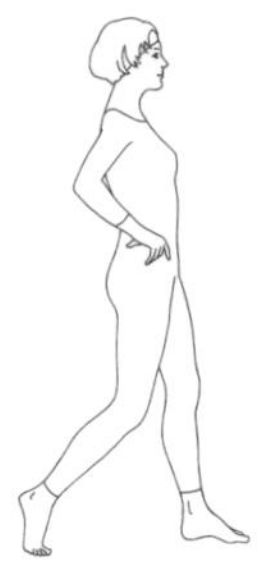

Standing hip flexor

STRETCH #23

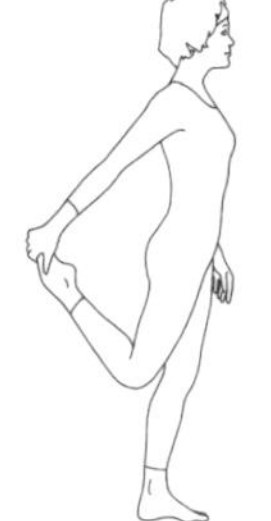

Standing quad stretch (quads and hip flexors)

STRETCH #20

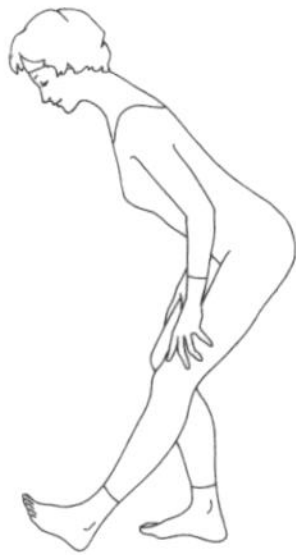

Standing hamstring stretch

STRETCH #30

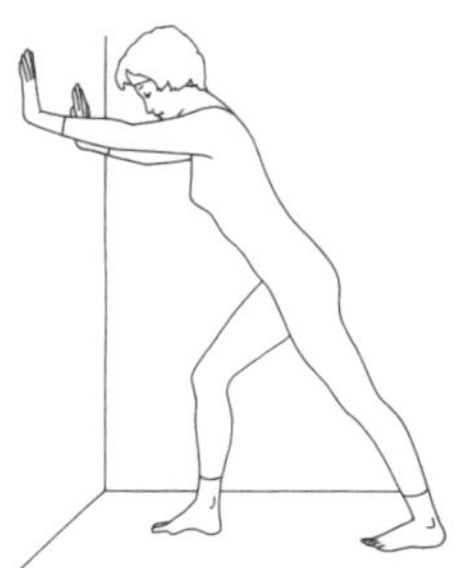

Standing calf stretch

STRETCH #39

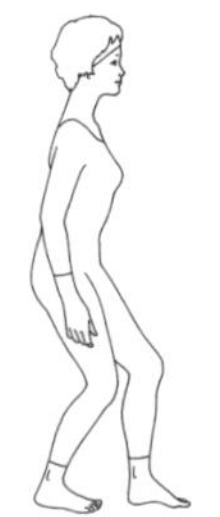

Standing soleus and Achilles stretch

STRETCH #42

Standing inner-thigh stretch

STRETCH #37

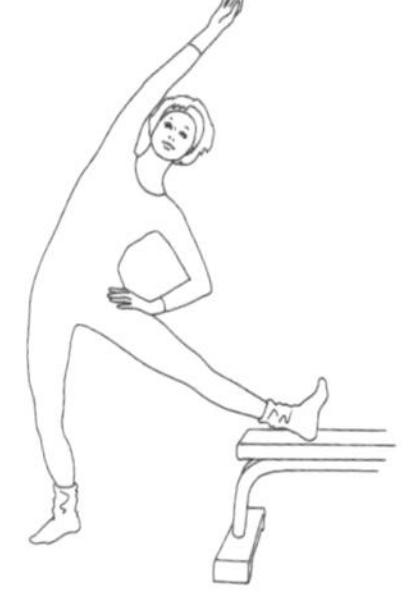

Overhead stretch (obliques and torso)

STRETCH #48

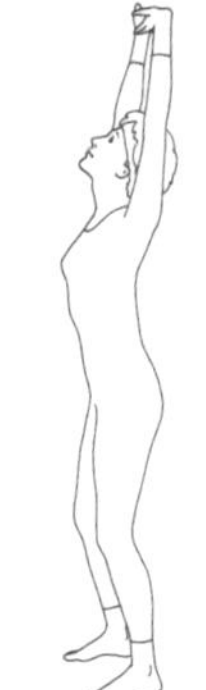

Side wrist pull (upper back)

STRETCH #53

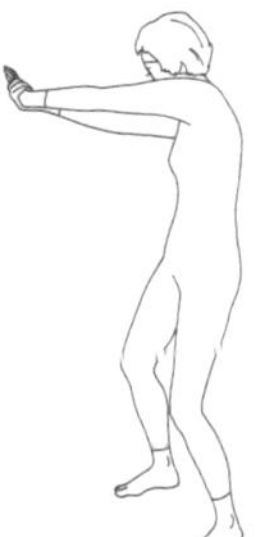

Hands behind your head (chest and front of shoulders)

STRETCH #57

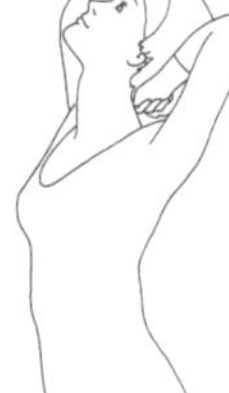

External rotator stretch (shoulders and arms)

STRETCH #62

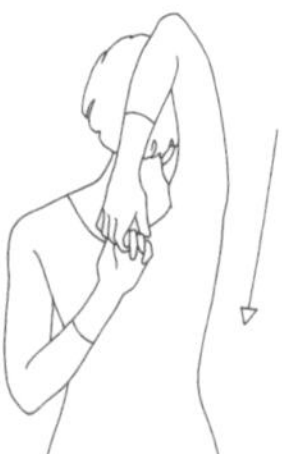

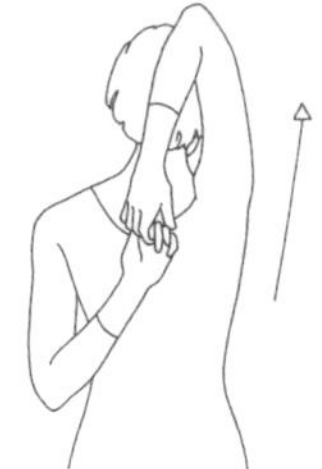

Internal rotator stretch (shoulders and arms)
STRETCH #63

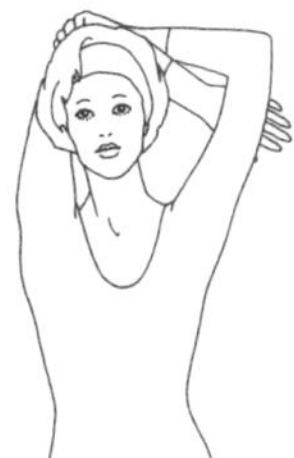

Triceps stretch (shoulders and arms)
STRETCH #64

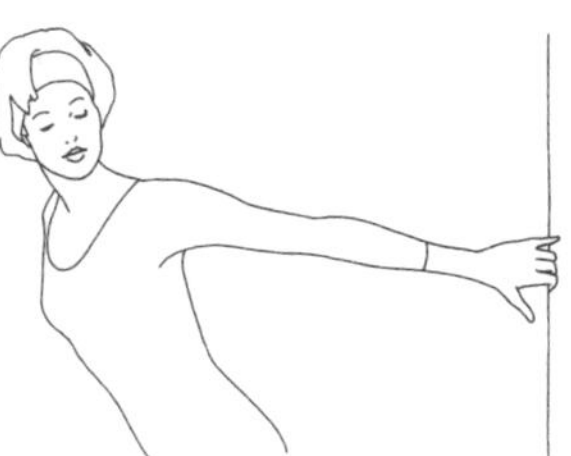

Biceps stretch (shoulders and arms)
STRETCH #65

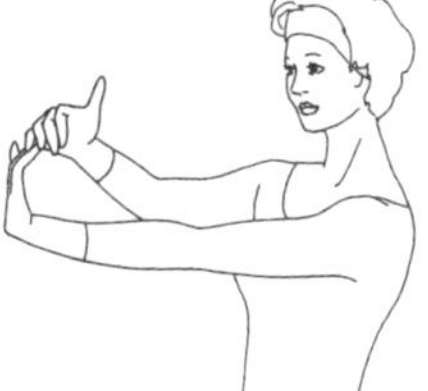

Wrist flexor stretch
STRETCH #69

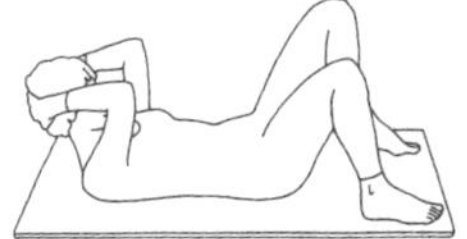

Back-of-the-neck stretch
STRETCH #66

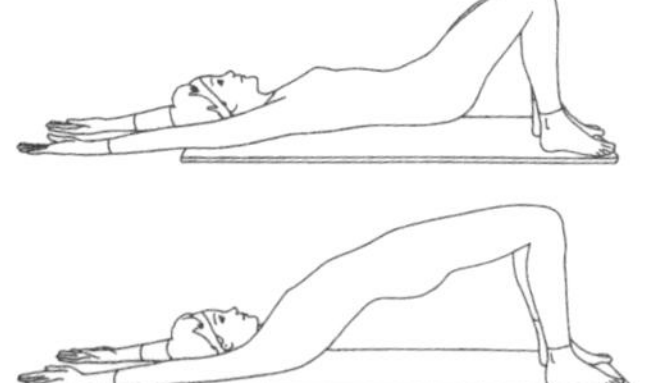

Pelvic tilt into bridge (lower back)
STRETCH #7

Hug knees to chest (lower back)
STRETCH #1

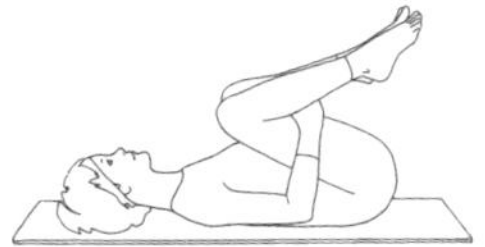

Ankle on the knee (buttocks, hips, and lower back)
STRETCH #14

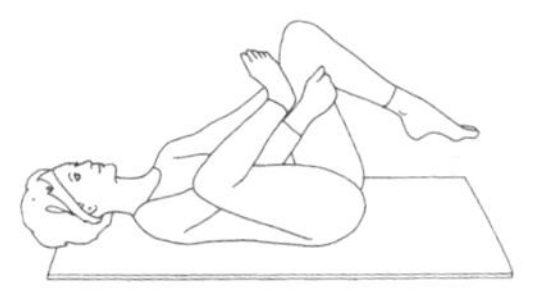

Knee across the body (buttocks, hips, and lower body)
STRETCH #13

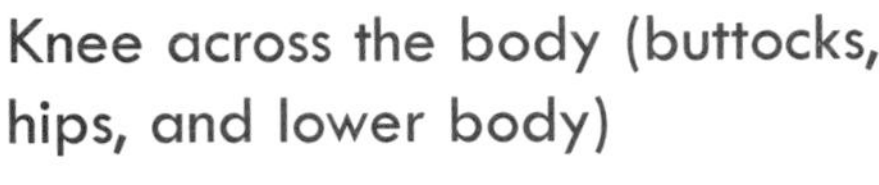

WALKING

Walking is such a popular form of exercise because it's easy to do and so much more forgiving on the joints than running. It's also an excellent aerobic workout, especially for people twenty or more pounds overweight. But to make walking a real workout, you have to walk like you're in a hurry and keep up that pace for 30 to 60 minutes. Walking uses only 50 to 60 percent of the calories you'd use if you ran the same distance.

Walking is also a great warm-up for stretching. If, like many people, you enjoy stretching before your walk to prepare yourself physically and mentally, do stretches #1–#8 but hold each one no longer than 10 seconds. Do them again after your walk, plus stretches #9–#14, holding each for 30 seconds. Improving your flexibility will lengthen and quicken your stride and minimize muscle soreness—especially in the hips, knees, and lower back.

While you walk, pay close attention to your stride. With every footfall, consciously land on your heel, roll to the ball of your foot, and use your toes to push off the pavement. Keep your knees springy and loose. Let your arms swing straight by your side in the slower part of your walk, and then bend and pump them as you speed up. Add hills to make the workout progressively harder. And since walking only works the lower body, be sure to add some form of upper-body strengthening—under the supervision of a qualified trainer or teacher if you're just learning how.

Standing calf stretch
STRETCH #39

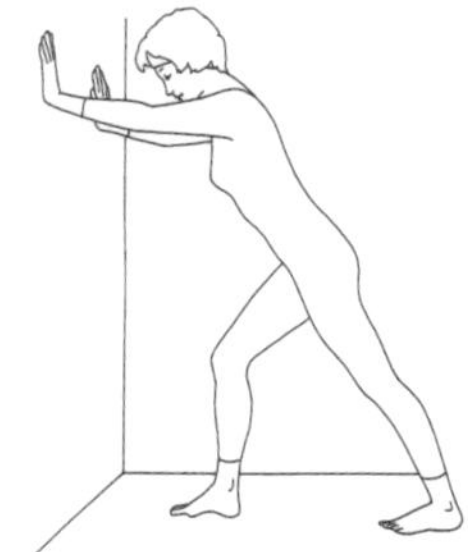

Standing soleus and Achilles stretch
STRETCH #42

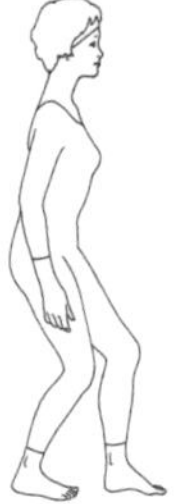

More advanced standing pelvic tilt (lower back)
STRETCH #9

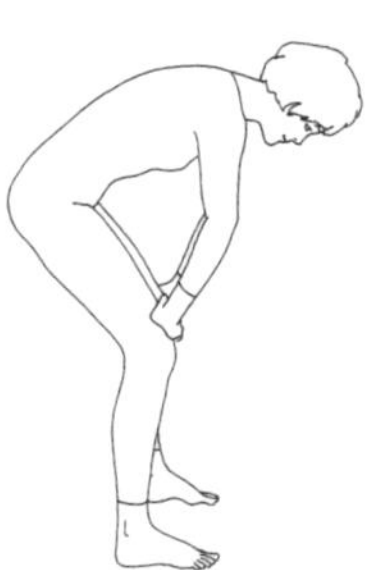

Standing quad stretch (quads and hip flexors)
STRETCH #20

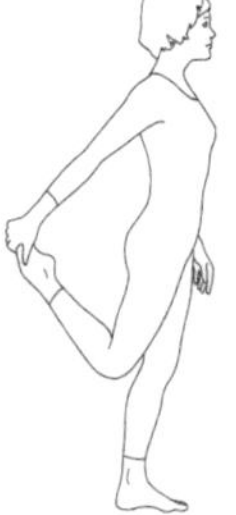

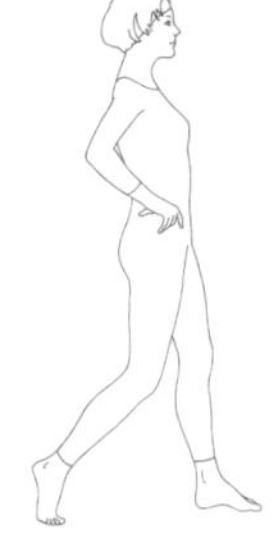

Standing hip flexor
STRETCH #23

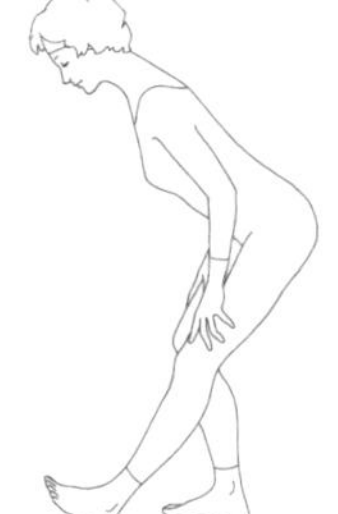

Standing hamstring stretch
STRETCH #30

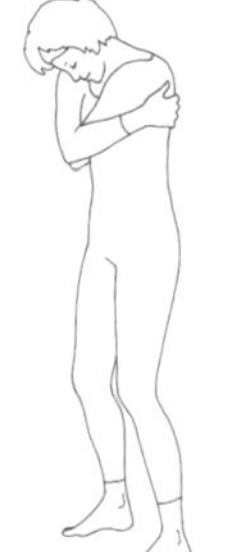

Hug yourself (upper back)
STRETCH #52

Arms low (chest)
STRETCH #58

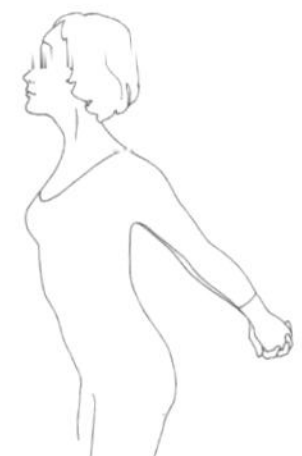

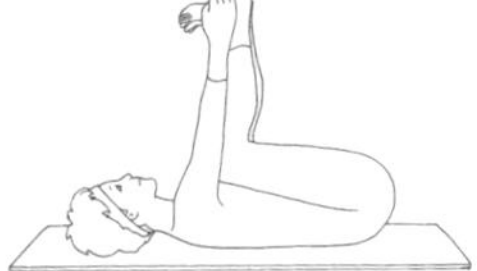

Erector spinae stretch (lower back)
STRETCH #2

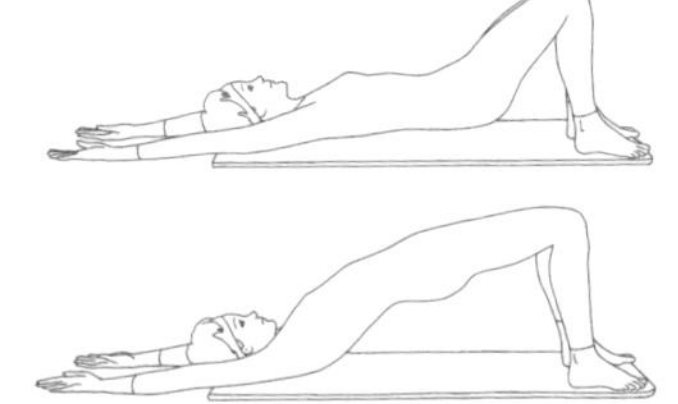

Pelvic tilt into bridge (lower back)
STRETCH #7

Full-body stretch (abdominals)
STRETCH #45

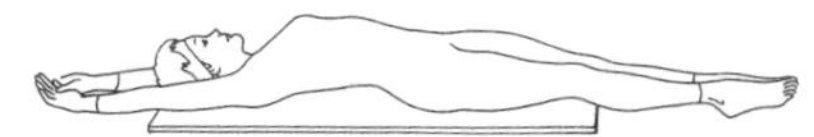

One knee to chest (buttocks, hips, and lower back)
STRETCH #12

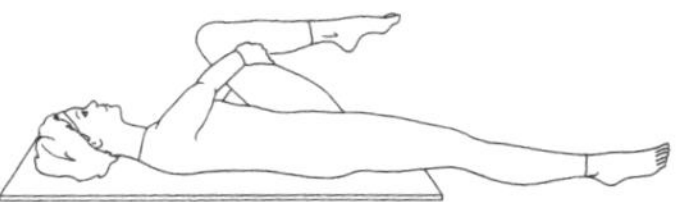

Ankle on the knee (buttocks, hips, and lower back)
STRETCH #14

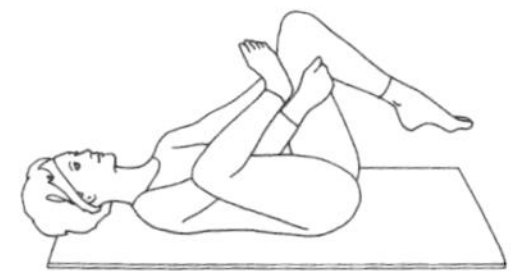

Knee across the body (buttocks, hips, and lower back)
STRETCH #13

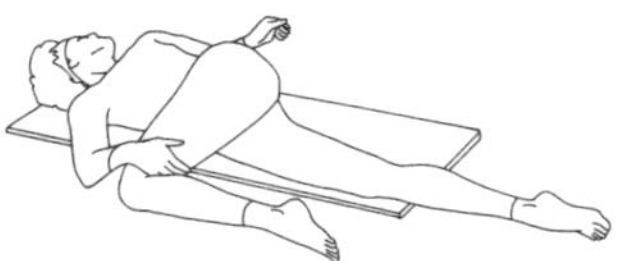

On-your-side quad stretch (quads and hip flexors)
STRETCH #19

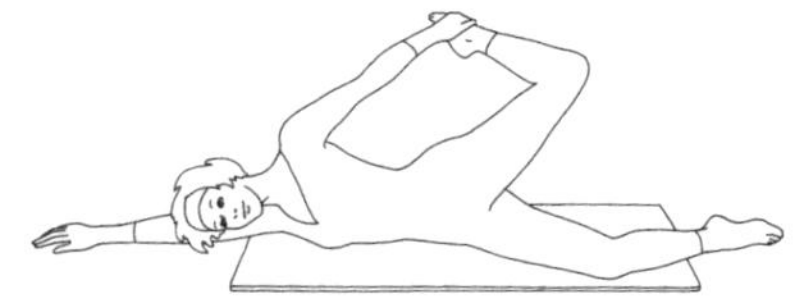

Side-lying groin stretch (inner thigh)
STRETCH #35

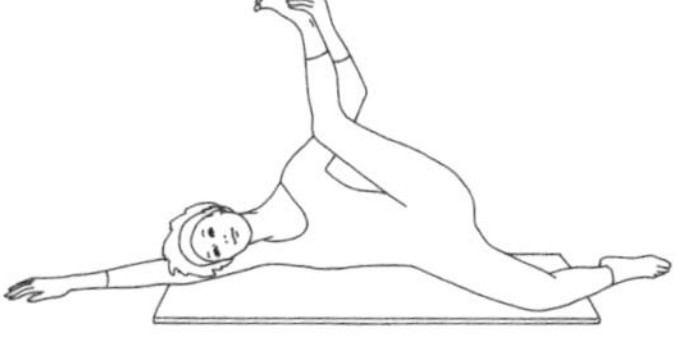

Side-lying floor stretch (outer hip and thigh)
STRETCH #31

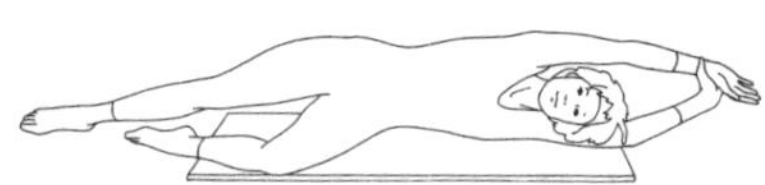

WEIGHT LIFTING

You probably already know that lifting weights can make you tighter (unless you stretch), but did you know that stretching can help make you stronger? When you lift weights, your muscles create a waste product called lactic acid (that "burning" sensation while you work out). Stretching flushes the lactic acid out of the muscles more quickly (both while you're exercising and after you're finished), so that you recover faster. Lifting also causes microtears in the muscles. In the one to four days after a workout, your muscles will get sore to the touch and become rigid as they heal. Flexible muscles, however, don't get as stiff or sore and therefore recover faster.

Stretching can also improve your weight-lifting form. Flexible muscles are better than stiff muscles at stabilizing other muscles and joints while you work specific body parts. And when your form is better, you cheat less, use your muscles more efficiently, get stronger, create a more pleasing physique, and have more fun at the gym!

Stretch when your muscles are fully engorged with blood—either just after your workout or between sets.

Erector spinae stretch (lower back)
STRETCH #2

Full-body stretch (abdominals)
STRETCH #45

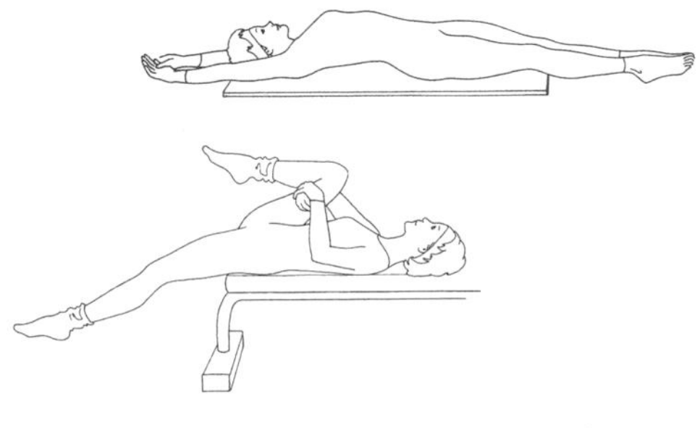

Bench hip flexor stretch
STRETCH #24

On-your-back quad stretch (quads and hip flexors)
STRETCH #17

Side-lying stretch on a bench (outer hip and thigh)

STRETCH #32

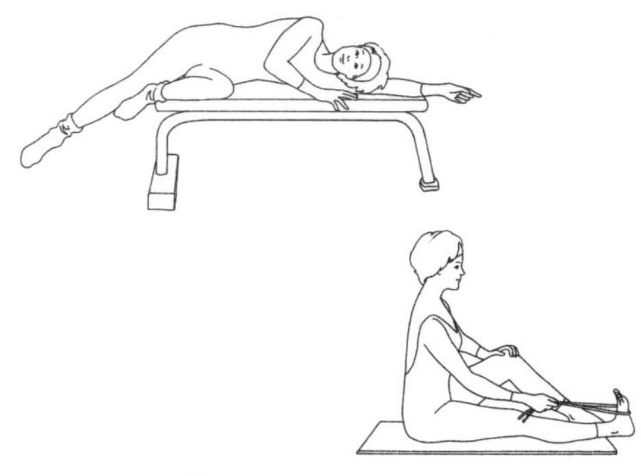

Floor or bench hamstring stretch

STRETCH #29

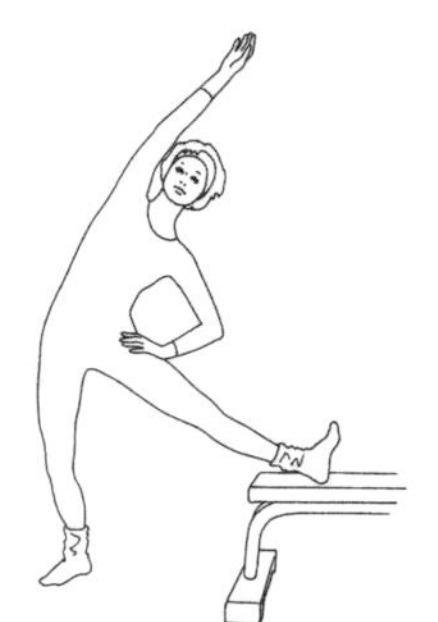

Standing inner-thigh stretch

STRETCH #37

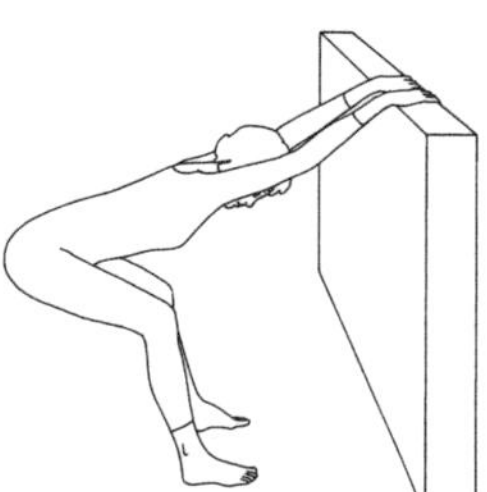

Sit-back stretch (upper back)

STRETCH #55

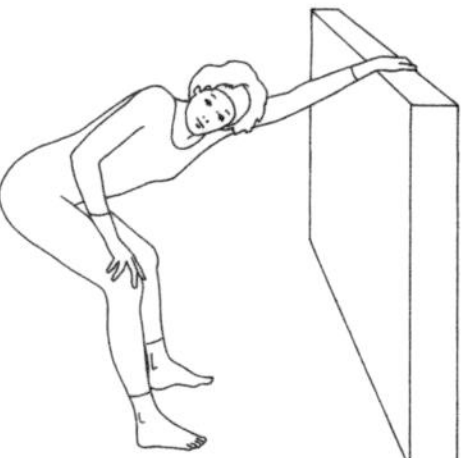

One-arm sit-back stretch (upper back)

STRETCH #56

The two-handed hang (hanging and inversion)

STRETCH #88

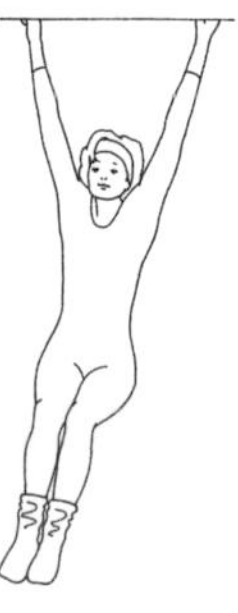

The one-handed hang (hanging and inversion)

STRETCH #89

The hyperextension-bench stretch (hanging and inversion)

STRETCH #90

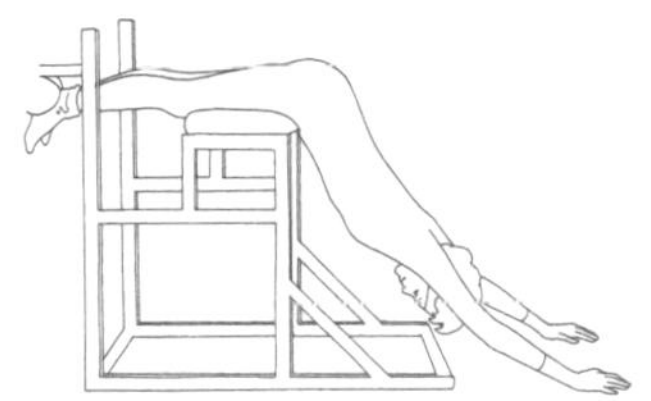

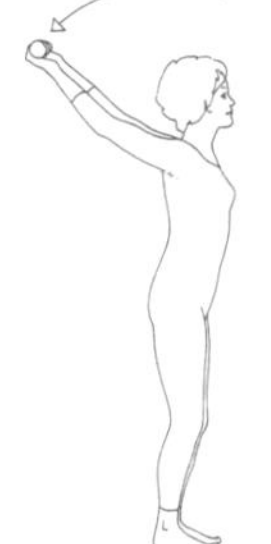

Chest and front-of-shoulder stretch (pole)

STRETCH #81

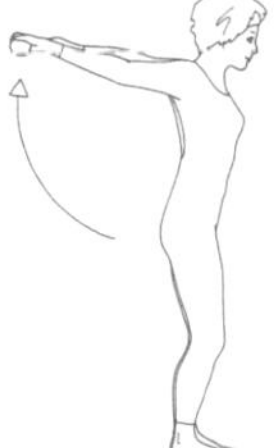

Round-the-world shoulder stretch (pole)

STRETCH #82

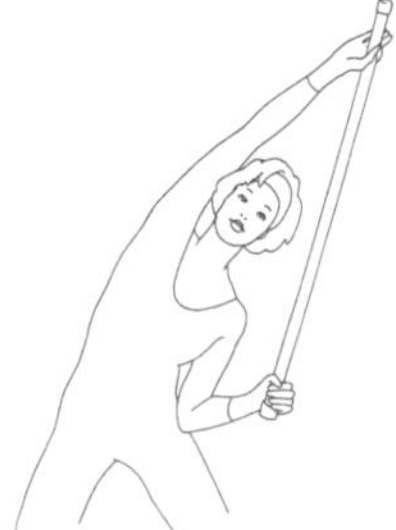

Side torso stretch (pole)

STRETCH #83

Hug a pole
STRETCH #84

External rotator stretch (shoulders and arms)
STRETCH #62

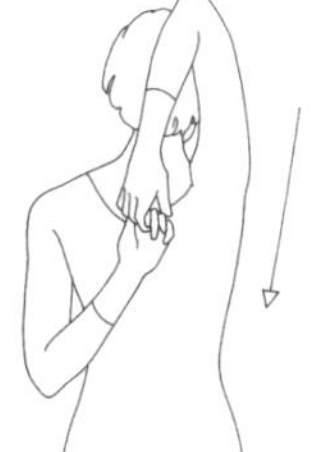

Internal rotator stretch (shoulders and arms)
STRETCH #63

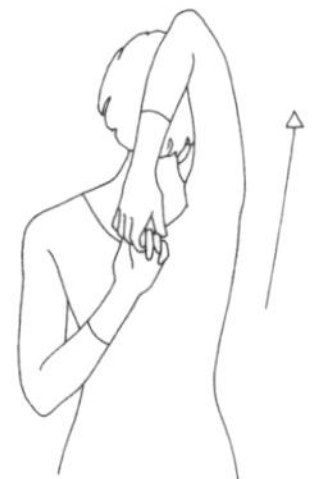

Triceps stretch (shoulders and arms)
STRETCH #64

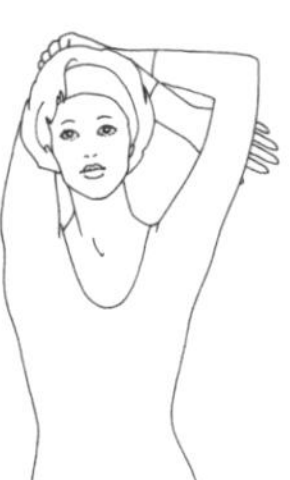

Biceps stretch (shoulders and arms)
STRETCH #65

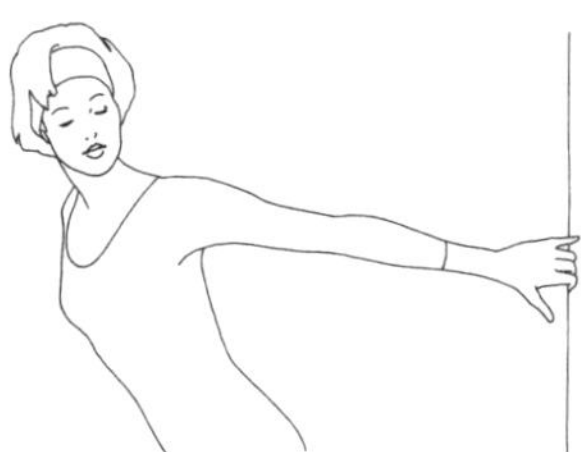

WINDSURFING

Although people who are good at it make it look easy, windsurfing can be difficult—especially when you are learning. All windsurfers need balance, quick reflexes, all-over strength (especially in the lower back and forearms), and head-to-toe flexibility. But beginners need even more since they wipe out a lot, have to pull the sail out of the water, and don't yet know how to perform the subtle moves that make windsurfing fluid and fun.

Good muscle stability is a must in this sport because the wind and water constantly force you to shift your center of balance. You also lean a lot—forward to lift the sail and back to ride the wind. You use the upper torso and arms to maneuver the sail, the abdominal muscles and lower back to lean backward, the legs to shift your weight, and the feet to grip the board. (When you lean forward to pull the sail, you shouldn't round your back. Bend your knees and arch your lower back as in a squatting position, then sit back into your hips and heels and be patient.)

If you like to stretch before you sail away, you can do these stretches gently, holding each for 10 seconds. The following stretches work best when your muscles are warm, after windsurfing or on days out of the water. Hold each position for 30 seconds.

Remember, it can get dangerous out on the water. Before you head out on your own, be sure you know what you're doing—have some lessons under your belt. Wear a flotation vest even if you think you're a strong swimmer and never go windsurfing without telling someone where you're going and how long you'll be.

Erector spinae stretch (lower back)

STRETCH #2

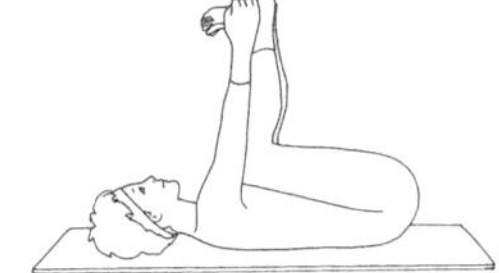

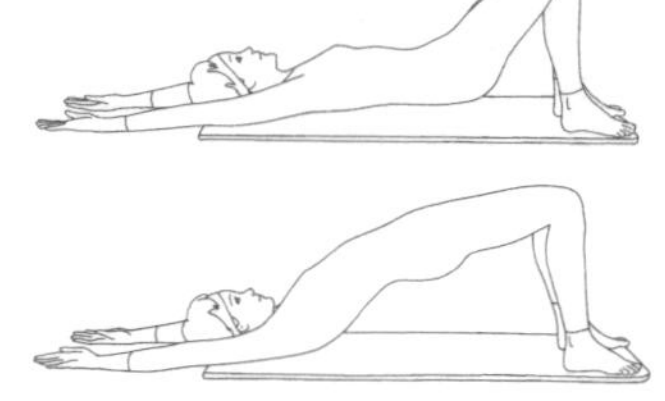

Pelvic tilt into bridge (lower back)
STRETCH #7

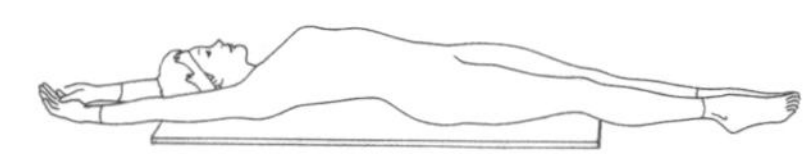

Full-body stretch (abdominals)
STRETCH #45

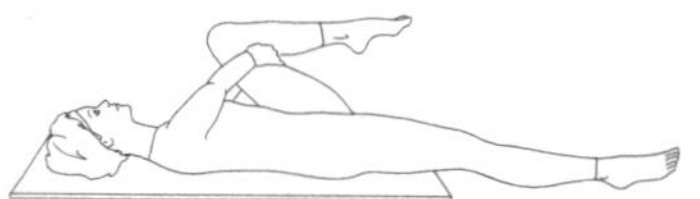

One knee to chest (buttocks, hips, and lower back)
STRETCH #12

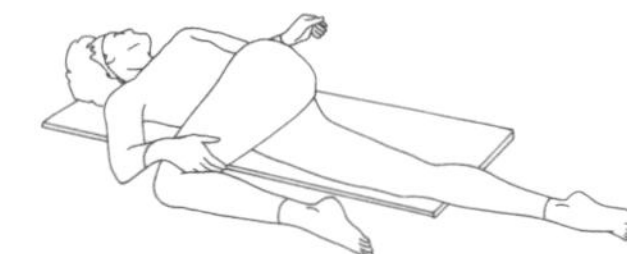

Knee across the body (buttocks, hips, and lower back)
STRETCH #13

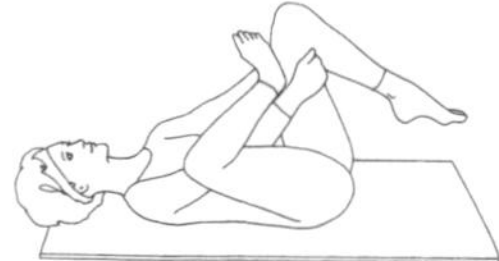

Ankle on the knee (buttocks, hips, and lower back)
STRETCH #14

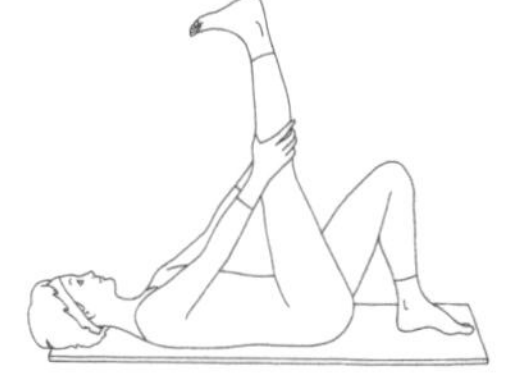

Leg-up hamstring stretch
STRETCH #27

Supine calf stretch (calves and Achilles)
STRETCH #40

Toe grab and spread (ankles and feet)
STRETCH #74

Back-of-the-neck stretch
STRETCH #66

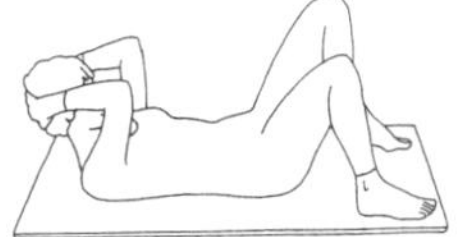

Side-lying groin stretch (inner thigh)
STRETCH #35

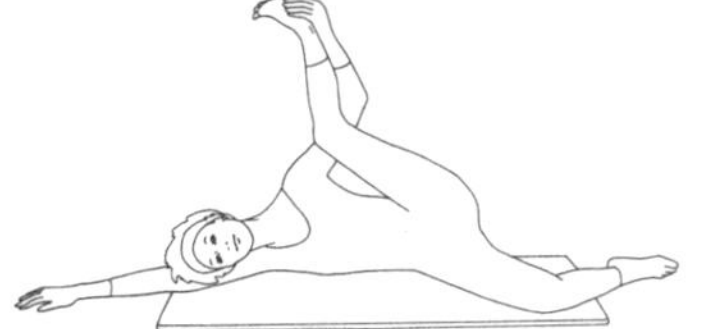

On-your-side quad stretch (quads and hip flexors)
STRETCH #19

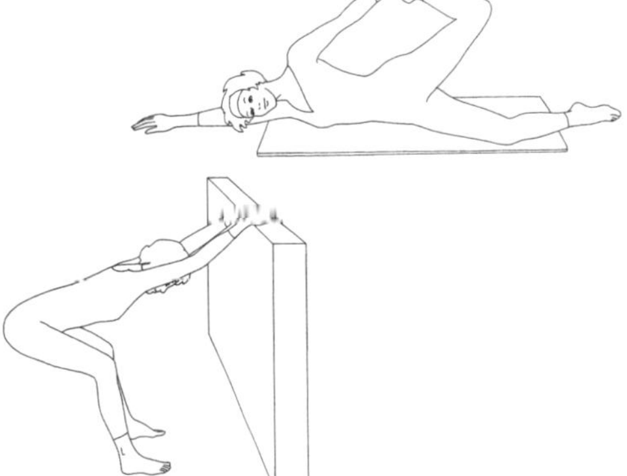

Sit-back stretch (upper back)
STRETCH #55

One-arm sit-back stretch (upper back)
STRETCH #56

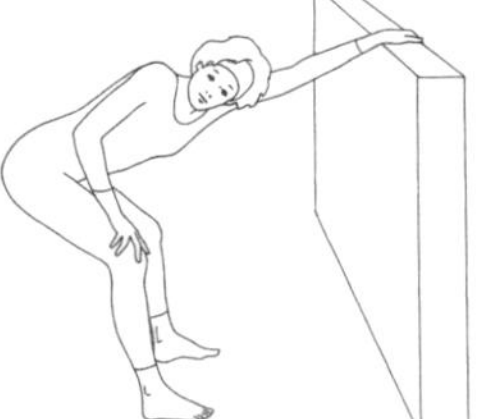

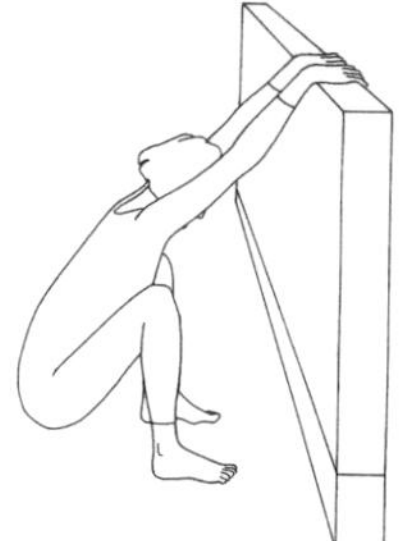

The full squat (lower back)

STRETCH #11

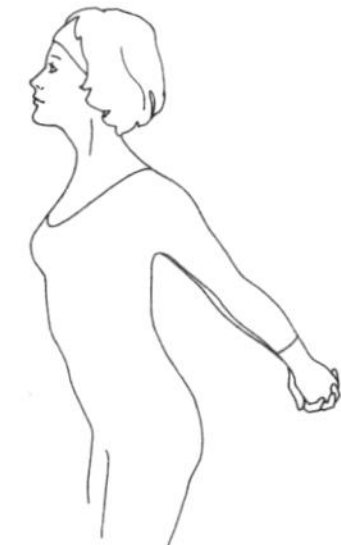

Arms low (chest)

STRETCH #58

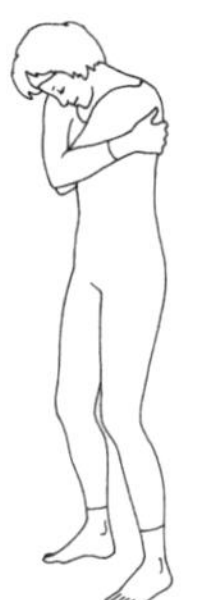

Hug yourself (upper back)

STRETCH #52

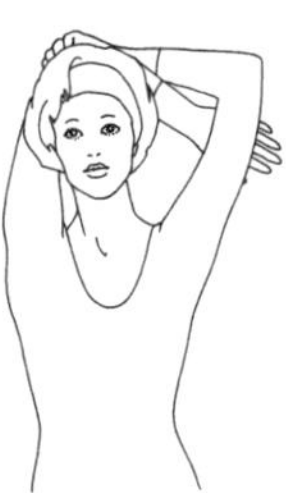

Triceps stretch (shoulders and arms)

STRETCH #64

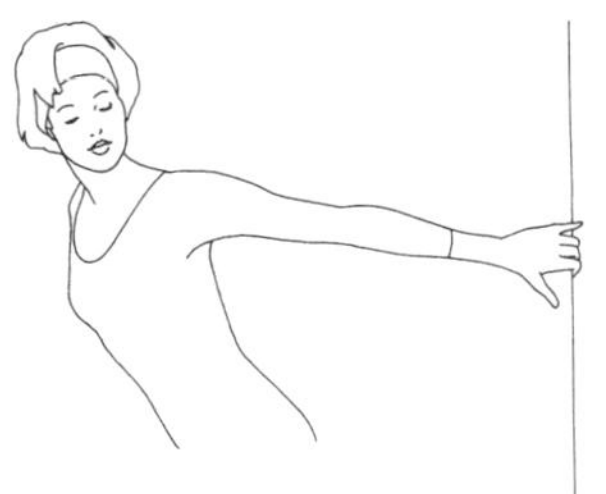

Biceps stretch (shoulders and arms)
STRETCH #65

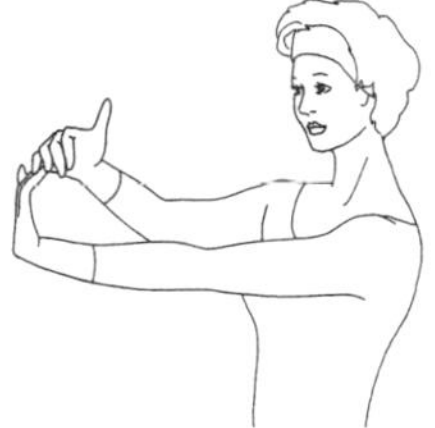

Wrist flexor stretch
STRETCH #69

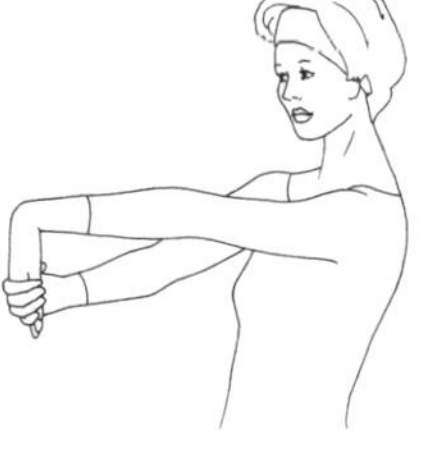

Wrist extensor stretch
STRETCH #70

STRETCHING DURING PREGNANCY

THANKS TO A HORMONE CALLED RELAXIN, PREGNANT WOMEN USUALLY BECOME MORE FLEXIBLE THAN THEY WERE BEFORE THEY GOT PREGNANT. IT SEEMS THAT MOTHER NATURE HAS VIRTUALLY "WIRED" WOMEN TO STRETCH DURING THIS TIME. ALL THIS FLEXIBILITY SERVES TWO PURPOSES FOR PREGNANCY AND CHILDBIRTH: NORMALLY, WHEN A MUSCLE OR ORGAN IS STRETCHED AS FAR AS THE UTERUS MUST STRETCH, IT CRAMPS. IF THIS WERE TO HAPPEN TO THE UTERUS, THE PREGNANCY WOULD TERMINATE. RELAXIN PREVENTS THIS. RELAXIN ALSO SOFTENS THE CONNECTIVE TISSUE IN THE PELVIS TO WIDEN THE BIRTH CANAL.

But there's a downside to this extra flexibility. Relaxin makes pregnant women somewhat "loose-jointed," which can make it easy for them to overstretch (this is also what gives pregnant women the "waddle"). Unlike muscle, overstretched connective tissue does not spring back to its original length, which leaves the body vulnerable to injury and arthritis later in life. Therefore, a pregnant woman who was flexible before pregnancy has to resist the urge to break new stretching records (especially during stretches to the most vulnerable joints, like the knees and spine) while pregnant and even for up to a year after giving birth, since relaxin circulates in the body for that long.

Don't get us wrong. Stretching is a wonderful form of exercise to do through pregnancy and beyond. It can ease all sorts of physical and mental discomforts: help a woman adjust to her body's shifting center of gravity, give her energy, and erase some of the stresses and fears associated with pending motherhood. It can also speed her recovery after childbirth.

If you are pregnant, you should approach stretching as you would any form of exercise. It is ideal to get in shape *before* you get pregnant; once you are pregnant, do your physical activities not to "get in shape" or keep your weight gain down but to maintain the highest level of health and safety for you and your baby. This isn't a time to try a new sport or break new records. You're better off maintaining your prepregnancy activities, tapering off as your body dictates. Of course, you should avoid activities like skating or soccer where you could fall or get hit; instead choose "minimal-impact" exercise that you enjoy and feels relatively easy to do. Walking and water aerobics are good cardiovascular choices. Strength training is a sensible option (and helps give you the strength to carry a growing child), but you shouldn't strain to lift heavy weights or use machines that force you onto your stomach or into uncomfortable positions. Respect what works for you and set aside what doesn't. Remember, each woman and each pregnancy is different.

Before you begin *any* exercise program, including stretching, be sure to get your doctor's permission. Get it again after delivery, before resuming your workouts, especially if you have had a cesarean section.

Some other important things you should know about pregnancy and exercise:

■ Don't get overheated.

Don't sit or stretch in a whirlpool, sauna, or steam room. When doing aerobic exercise, avoid working at too high a heart rate (this avoids overheating and overexerting). Use the following heart-rate guidelines for your age group: under 20: 140–55; 20–29: 135–50; 30–39: 130–45; and over 40: 125–40.

■ Drink more water than you think you need.

Dehydration can cause an early labor. Drink water before, during, and after exercise—even a stretching workout. Once you're thirsty, you're already somewhat dehydrated.

■ Eat every few hours, even if you don't feel like it and even if it's just a snack.

When you're pregnant, you consume three hundred more calories per day than before. Add exercise, and you'll need even more. Several small meals throughout the day can keep your energy up and will nourish your baby.

■ Stop exercising immediately and call your doctor if you experience any pain, bleeding, contractions, dizziness, nausea, or numbness.

■ Don't lie on your back for long, especially after the first trimester.

This position reduces blood flow to the uterus. The best postures for exercise and stretching while pregnant are standing, seated upright, or supported, forward-leaning stretches, either standing or on your hands and knees.

■ Be mindful of your wrists.

Your extremities usually swell during pregnancy. This can affect the nerves in your wrists and cause carpal tunnel syndrome. Avoid putting excessive weight on your wrists (especially during stretches on your hands and knees) if this causes pain.

Seated lower-back stretch
STRETCH #3

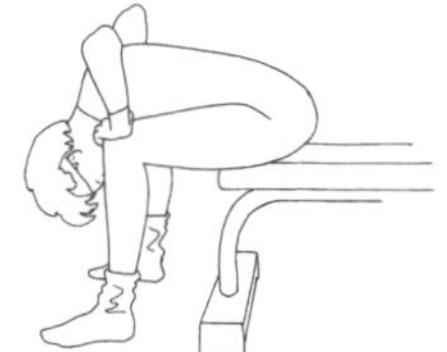

Seated or standing twist (lower back)
STRETCH #4

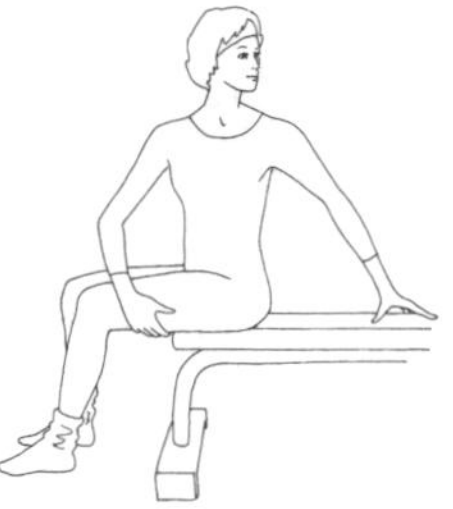

Floor or bench hamstring stretch
STRETCH #29

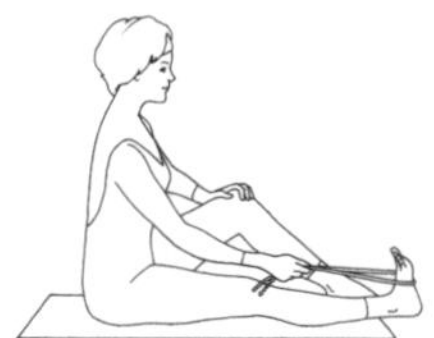

Hang over a chair (inner thigh)
STRETCH #36

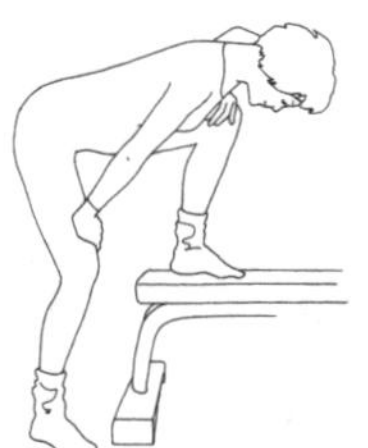

Standing pelvic tilt (lower back)
STRETCH #8

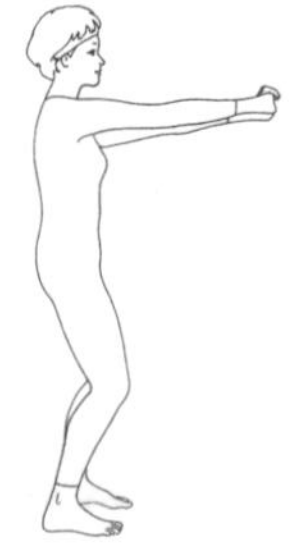

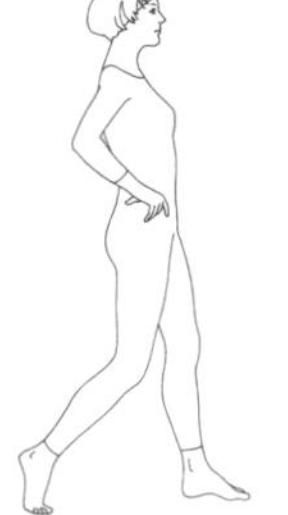

Standing hip flexor
STRETCH #23

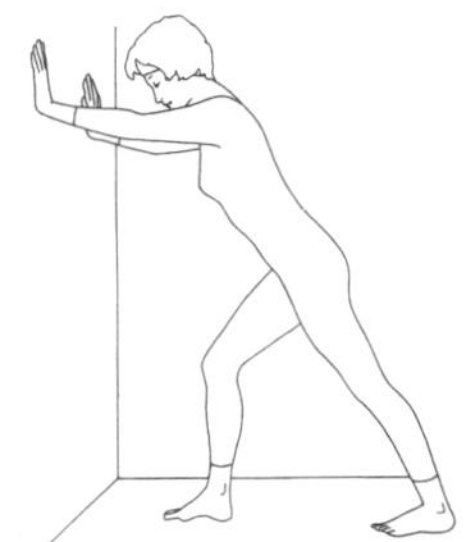

Standing calf stretch
STRETCH #39

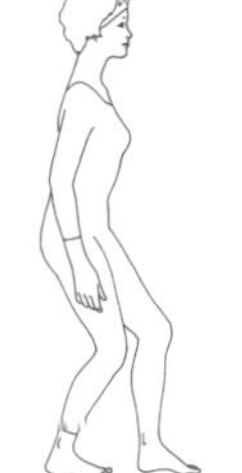

Standing soleus and Achilles stretch
STRETCH #42

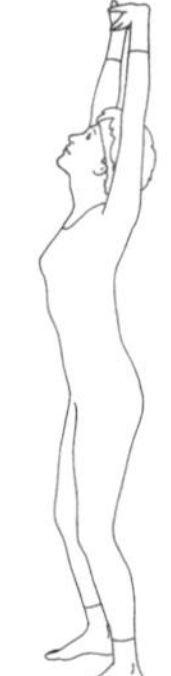

Overhead stretch (obliques and torso)
STRETCH #48

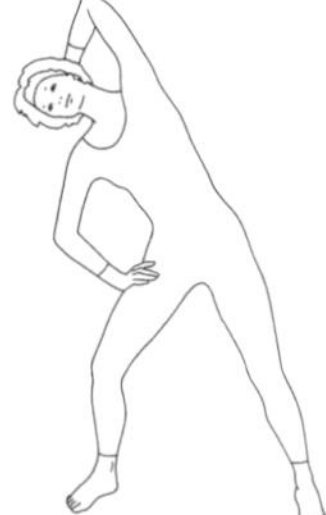

Standing lateral stretch (obliques and torso)
STRETCH #49

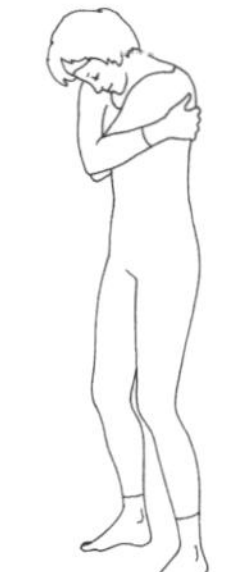

Hug yourself (upper back)
STRETCH #52

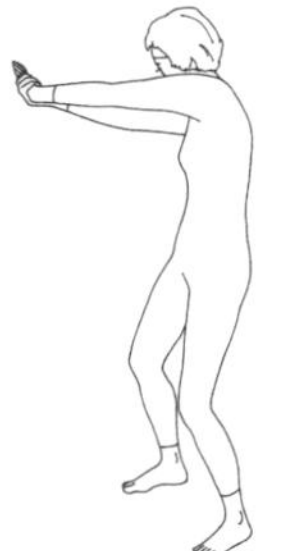

Side wrist pull (upper back)
STRETCH #53

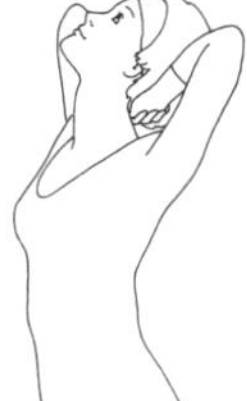

Hands behind your head (chest and front of shoulders)
STRETCH #57

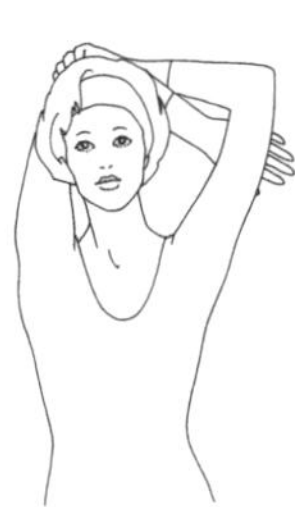

Triceps stretch (shoulders and arms)
STRETCH #64

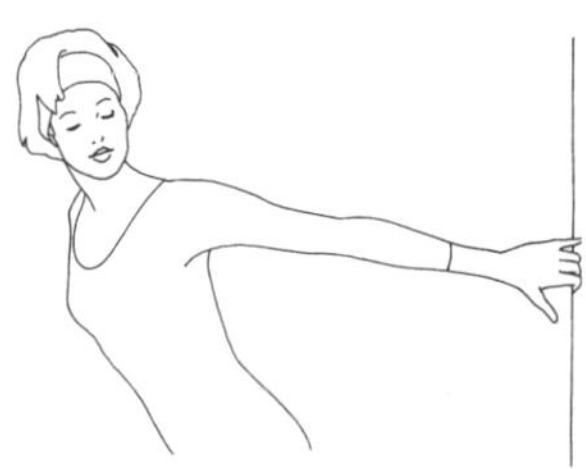

Biceps stretch (shoulders and arms)
STRETCH #65

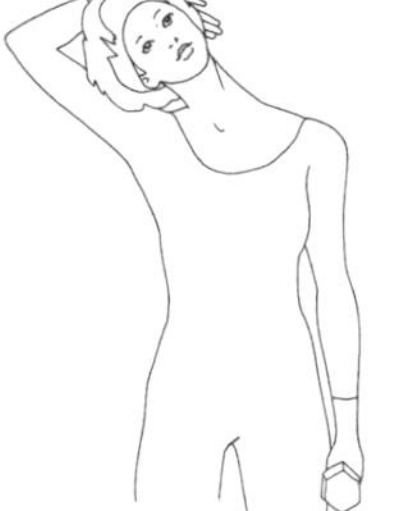

Lateral neck stretch
STRETCH #67

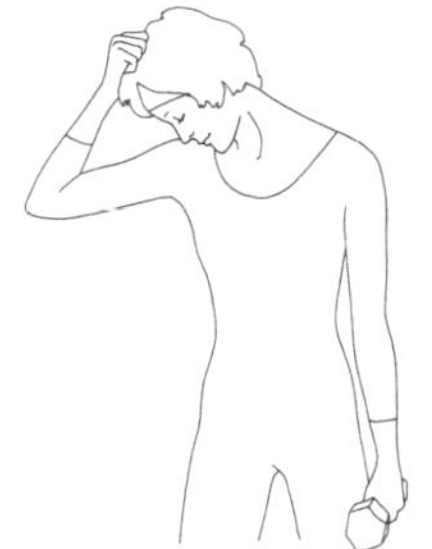

Oblique extensor stretch (neck)
STRETCH #68

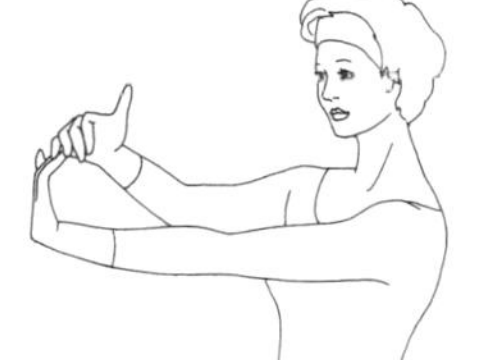

Wrist flexor stretch
STRETCH #69

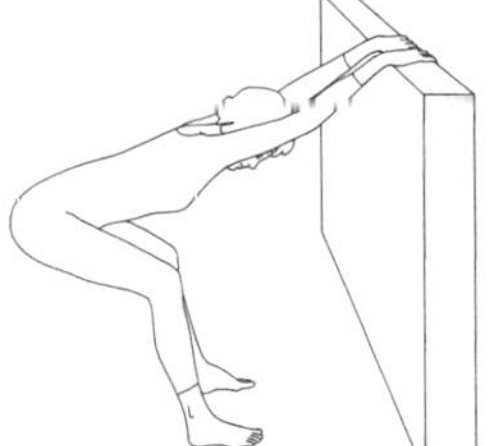

Sit-back stretch (upper back)
STRETCH #55

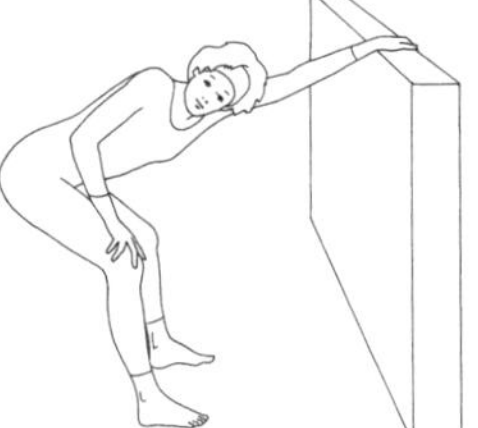

One-arm sit-back stretch (upper back)
STRETCH #56

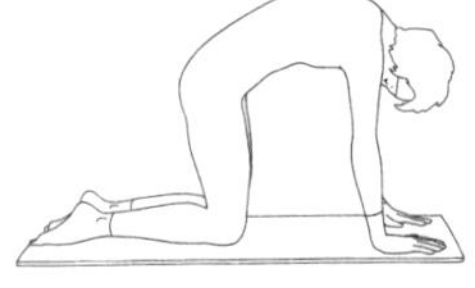

Cat stretch (lower back)
STRETCH #5

All-fours twist (upper back)
STRETCH #54

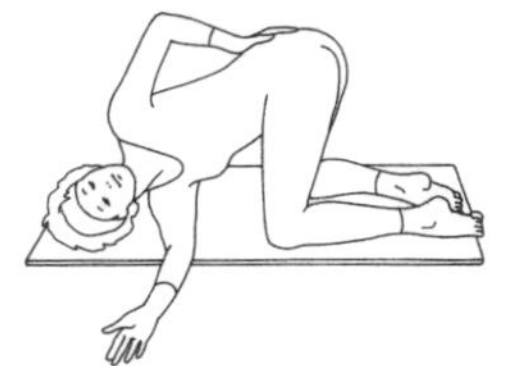

On-your-side quad stretch (quads and hip flexors)
STRETCH #19

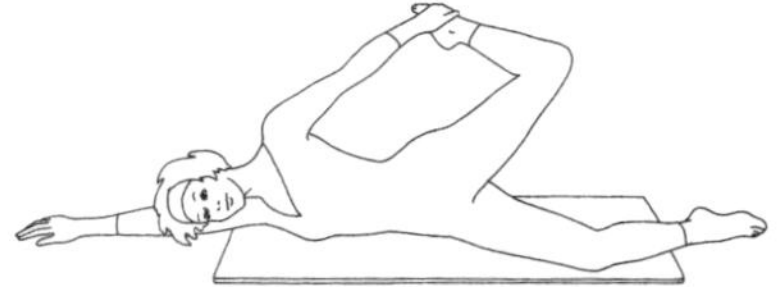

Side-lying floor stretch (outer hip and thigh)
STRETCH #31

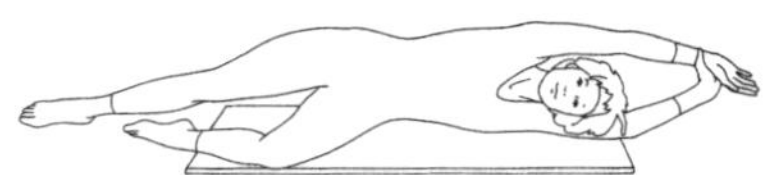

Side-lying groin stretch (inner thigh)
STRETCH #35

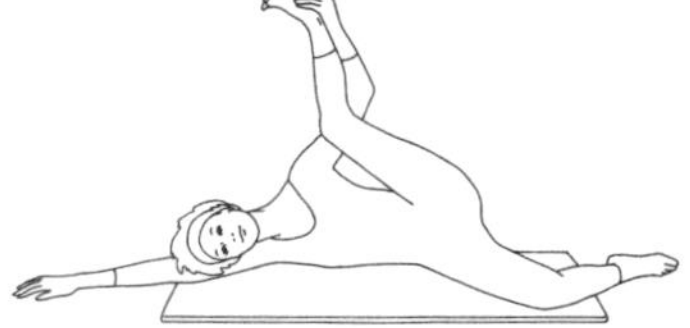

Seated butterfly stretch (inner thigh)
STRETCH #34

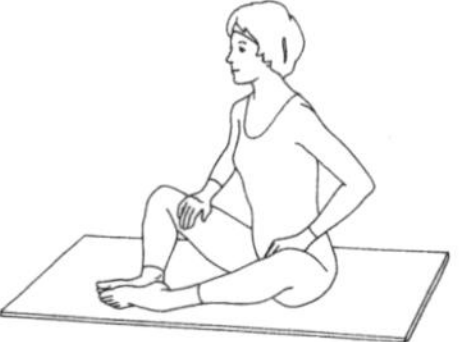

BIBLIOGRAPHY

Alter, Judy, *Stretch and Strengthen*, New York: Houghton Mifflin, 1992.

Alter, Michael J., *Science of Flexibility*, 2d edition, Champaign, Ill.: Human Kinetics Publishing, 1996.

Alter, Michael J., *Sports Stretch*, 2d edition, Champaign, Ill.: Human Kinetics Publishing, 1997.

American Council on Exercise, *Aerobics Instructor Manual*, 2d edition, San Diego, Cal.: American Council on Exercise Publication, 1997.

American Council on Exercise, *Personal Trainer Manual*, 2d edition, San Diego, Cal.: American Council on Exercise Publication, 1996.

Anderson, Bob, *Stretching*, Bolinas, Cal.: Shelter Publications, 1980.

Black, Sarah, *The Supple Body: The Way to Fitness, Strength, and Flexibility*, New York: Macmillan, 1997.

Fitness magazine, Editors of, with Karen Andes, *The Complete Book of Fitness: Mind, Body, Spirit*, New York: Three Rivers Press, 1999.

Kurz, Thomas, M.Sc., *Stretching Scientifically: A Guide to Flexibility Training*, 3d edition, Island Pond, Vt.: Stadion Publishing Company, 1994.

Martins, Peter, *The New York City Ballet Workout: 50 Stretches and Exercises Anyone Can Do for a Strong, Graceful, and Sculpted Body*, New York: William Morrow and Company, 1997.

Robinson, Lynn, Gordon Thompson, and Piers Chandler, *Body Control the Pilates Way*, London, England: Boxtree, 1997.

Wharton, Jim, and Phil Wharton, *The Whartons' Stretch Book: Featuring the Breakthrough Method of Active-Isolated Stretching*, New York: Times Books, 1996.

I N D E X

G

H

I

T